Continuous Quality Improvement for Health Information Management

Jennifer I. Cofer, RRA
Hugh P. Greeley

Opus Communications
Marblehead, Massachusetts

Continuous Quality Improvement for Health Information Management is published by Opus Communications.

Copyright 1998 by Opus Communications, Inc.

All rights reserved. Printed in the United States of America. 5 4 3 2 1

ISBN 1-57839-039-7

Opus Communications provides information resources for the healthcare industry. A selected listing of other newsletters and books is found in the back of this book. Arrangements can be made for quantity discounts.

Jennifer I. Cofer, Executive Publisher, Author
Hugh P. Greeley, Author
Rob Stuart, Publisher
Kristen Woods, Executive Editor
David Beardsley, Managing Editor
Jean St. Pierre, Art Director
Mike Mirabello, Graphic Artist
Thomas Philbrook, Cover Designer

Advice given is general. Readers should consult professional counsel for specific legal, ethical, or clinical questions. Opus Communications is not affiliated in any way with the Joint Commission on Accreditation of Healthcare Organizations.

For more information on this or other Opus Communications publications, contact:

Opus Communications
PO Box 1168
Marblehead, MA 01945
Telephone: 800/650-6787 or 781/639-1872
Fax: 800/639-8511 or 781/639-2982
E-mail: customer_service@opuscomm.com

Visit the Opus Communications World Wide Web site: www.opuscomm.com

Table of Contents

Table of Contents

In an age of mega-mergers and far-flung healthcare networks, many organizations face the difficult task of integrating systems and standardizing procedures across different locations and care settings. Here's how one network of ambulatory clinics used CQI to confront that challenge.

Healthcare organizations spend a lot of time collecting data—so much, in fact, that they may have little time available for effective analysis. Furthermore, reliance on chart review as a data-collection tool can generate a mountain of chart requests for HIM staff to process. It's a dilemma that a CQI team at this Texas hospital decided to address.

Taking a proactive approach to CQI often allows organizations to spot and correct problems in their earliest stages—before they become damaging crises. A case in point is this Florida-based hospital network that nipped a delinquent-records trend in the bud.

It is, perhaps, the most difficult accreditation requirement for home-care agencies to meet: ensuring that doctors sign orders and plans of care within the timeframe set by the state and the JCAHO. Thanks to a committed CQI team, this South Carolina agency saw its on-time return rate increase eight-fold in a single year.

Case-Study Figures (Chapter 5)

Ambulatory Clinics Standardize Documentation and Posting *101*

About the Authors

Jennifer I. Cofer, **RRA,** is the founder and executive publisher of Opus Communications, which publishes *Medical Records Briefing, Briefings on* JCAHO, and many other books and newsletters. She is also practice director for health information management at The Greeley Company. Ms. Cofer has developed survey preparation tools and techniques for information management, lectures and consults on survey preparation and HIM-related accreditation standards, and serves as an advisor on medical-records documentation and information management.

In 1991, Ms. Cofer served as president of the American Health Information Management Association. She has also served as that organization's director of communications and professional practices, and as editor of the *Journal of* AMRA (now *Journal of* AHIMA). In 1993, AHIMA presented Ms. Cofer with the Edna K. Huffman award for her literary pursuits. Ms. Cofer recently edited the tenth edition of the renowned Huffman textbook, now titled *Health Information Management.*

Hugh P. Greeley is the chairman and founder of The Greeley Company. Mr. Greeley has participated as a faculty member in over 2,500 seminars on continuous quality improvement, medical staff organization, credentialing, trustee responsibility, antitrust, accreditation, or other related subjects.

Mr. Greeley was a member of the board and professional affairs committee of Deaconess-Incarnate Word Health System in St. Louis, Missouri. He is a partner in The Credentialling Institute, an educational institute located in Pittsburgh, Pennsylvania, and he serves on the faculties of the Estes Park Institute and the American College of Physician Executives. Prior to forming The Greeley Company, Mr. Greeley held a number of positions with the Joint Commission on Accreditation of Healthcare Organizations, InterQual, Inc., and Kenosha Hospital Medical Center.

Mr. Greeley is a contributing editor to many healthcare journals and the author of numerous books and articles.

Acknowledgments

Thanks to Darice Grzybowski, Mary Mike Pavoni, Mary Radley, Patrice Spath, and Tella Marie Williams for their advice and input. Thanks to Jim Braden for his introduction, and to Larry Dunham, Pam Haines, Debbie Hepburn, and LaVonne Wieland for their help with and work on the case studies. Thanks also to Deborah Arseneaux, Betty Biles, Mary Brandt, Nancy Davis, Karen Frazer, Julie-Leah Harding, Carl Hula, Lucy Limones, Brenda Nicholson, Lesley Paulsen, Sheela Rao, Karen Williams Reinhold, and Jack Segal.

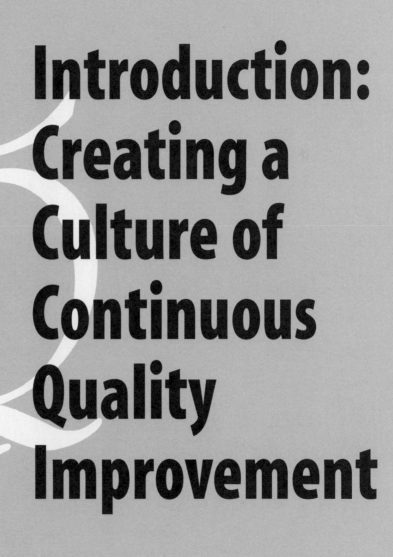

Introduction: Creating a Culture of Continuous Quality Improvement

Introduction: Creating a Culture of Continuous Quality Improvement
by James H. Braden, MBA

Like healthcare in general, health information management (HIM) is a field in flux. For HIM professionals, this environment of change is both challenging and exciting. To progress and succeed, we must constantly reengineer our processes and organizations to better address customer expectations, which are increasing noticeably. We can no longer be satisfied with looking at continuous quality improvement (CQI) simply as a tactic for retrospective evaluation. Rather, we must weave CQI into the cultural fabric of our profession, making it a prospective tool and an integral part of our departments and our processes. We can no longer afford to think in terms of "moments of change." Rather, we must embrace true CQI by creating mechanisms that encourage ongoing evolution—supported by data analysis—and that are driven by an empowered, entrepreneurial staff. Certainly, that was the intent of experts like Deming, Juran, and Joiner, whose thinking on quality and management laid the foundation for CQI.

Today's HIM departments are asked to do more with less: to deliver higher quality products at a lower unit cost; to process, retain, and disseminate more information with fewer human resources. Consequently, many HIM departments now view CQI as an expendable activity; when push comes to shove, they put improvement programs "on the shelf" and focus on meeting the most immediate demands of their customers. Although that approach might produce the desired bottom-line results, it ultimately jeopardizes quality and morale. It is critical that we consider an alternative approach. Rather than downsizing departments and asking the remaining staff to carry a bigger load (though that may be unavoidable in some instances), we should encourage workers to develop smarter long-term work habits and more efficient systems through CQI.

We can't afford to ignore CQI from an accreditation standpoint either. The Joint Commission on Accreditation of Healthcare Organizations (JCAHO) expects facilities to integrate improvement efforts and to create a CQI culture. The JCAHO views CQI as part and parcel to the mission of healthcare organizations, and its surveyors look for evidence that improvement functions are embedded and occur naturally within an organization.

But seeking to adopt true CQI means shifting our paradigms. It creates a context in which HIM management must view itself as working for the HIM staff, not the reverse. HIM managers must define the vision of a change-minded culture, role-model that vision, and remove the obstacles (real or perceived) to realizing it. However, we cannot be the agents of continuous improvement; nor can we single-handedly create a culture that embraces it. For CQI to take root in a department's culture, the entire staff must embrace and nurture it. What we need is an improvement process that is supported at the top but implemented and controlled from the bottom. That's a radical shift, which requires mutual trust and new lines of accountability.

At the University of Texas Medical Branch Hospitals and Clinics (UTMB), where I served as director of health information management for more than five years, we recognized the need for radical change in 1993. Over a period of 18 months, our department phased out a traditional pyramid-shaped management structure, in which top-level managers made decisions that lower-level employees acted upon like "good soldiers." We cut the layers of management between the director and the front-line staff from five to one and established 18 self-directed work teams, each with a broad mandate to shape and govern its primary departmental functions.

To avoid having teams become isolated fiefdoms, we created mechanisms that encourage interdependency. For instance, poor performance by one team affects the performance reviews of all employees—whether they "serve" on that team or not. As a result, teams share resources, including staff, which helps to alleviate the pressures of short-term deadlines and, more significantly, prompts spontaneous, ongoing questioning of systems and processes. This questioning can trigger significant long-term change and is a hallmark of CQI. Under this system, employees who are asked to "help out" have an interest in doing so, but they also have an interest in identifying opportunities for streamlining processes to reduce the likelihood that backlogs, logjams, and other work-flow issues arise again.

Our HIM teams have partnered with each other to reengineer many work processes. They begin with desired outcomes in mind, which they define based on the expectations of customers and constituents. Using the FADE (Focus, Analyze, Develop, Execute) approach to CQI (similar to the PDCA method discussed here, in Chapter 4), they redesign the work of our department to achieve those outcomes. When we introduced the team approach, for instance, our department, which receives about nine thousand loose reports per day, had 350 thousand unfiled reports. The loose-reports team set out to design a system that would eliminate the backlog and ensure that nothing went unfiled for more than 36 hours. The team succeeded, and has consistently met that 36-hour standard since November 1994.

Guaranteeing the autonomy and decision-making power of the HIM teams has been key to our approach. When we introduced the team concept, we ceremoniously tossed the department's procedures manual in the trash bin, telling staff they would no longer be told how to do their jobs or be held to specific productivity standards. Their work is driven only by the desired outcomes of our customers and, freed of bureaucratic barriers, they do whatever is necessary (provided it's legal and ethical) to achieve those outcomes. This approach facilitates the staff's ability to "think outside the box" and constantly refine their work processes.

The teams agree annually on customer-service outcomes, which are reflected in the department's annual business plan. And they've developed integrated monitoring mechanisms that provide an ongoing flow of data to measure their performance against those outcomes. The HIM department communicates this data graphically to all teams, and to our customer base. It's also posted on the department's Internet home page (UTMB.*edu/him/*) for all the world to see. Based on this data, teams make adjustments and monitor the results "on the fly." CQI is no longer viewed as an added task or responsibility; it is an integrated, instinctive part of everyone's job, and that enables us to achieve a level of performance that is both high and sustainable.

UTMB's way is not the only way. This book, *Continuous Quality Improvement for Health Information Management*, is designed to help HIM departments, professionals, and students adapt CQI to their work processes and cultures. It provides a solid introduction to CQI theories and tools, and discusses how to apply them in the demanding and data-rich HIM environment. In a series of compelling case studies, it explores how HIM departments have actually used CQI tools and techniques, with impressive results. Finally, it offers practical tips on how to introduce and maintain a CQI program in your organization.

James H. Braden, MBA, served as director of health information management at the 1,000-bed University of Texas Medical Branch, in Galveston, TX, from 1993 until 1998. He is now system director, health information management, at the Detroit Medical Center in Detroit, MI, an eight-hospital network with nearly 3,000 beds and that sees about 1.6 million outpatients each year.

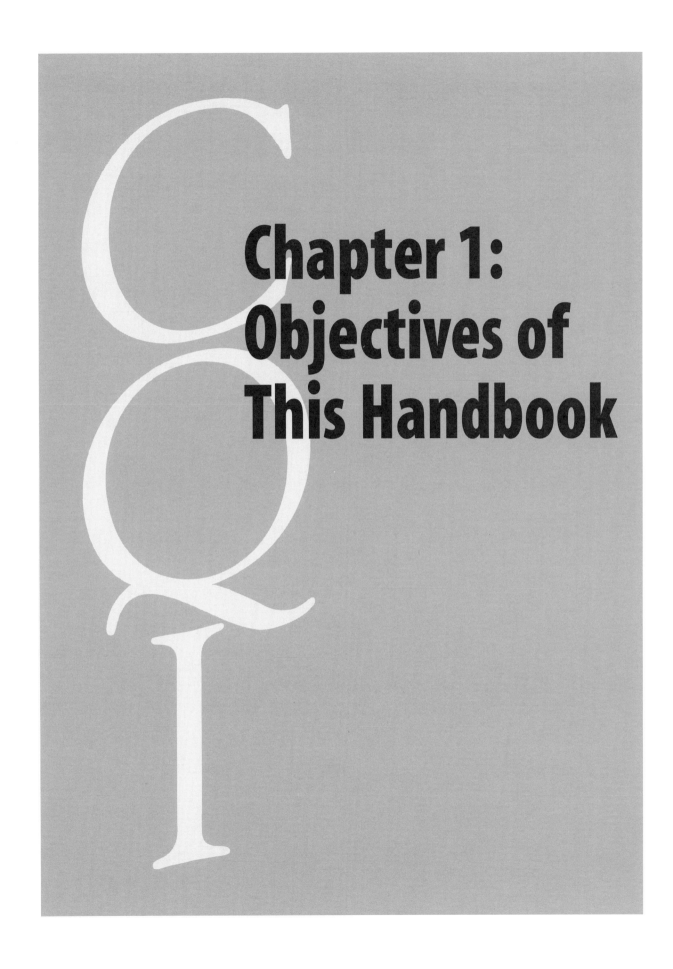

Chapter 1:
Objectives of
This Handbook

Chapter 1: Objectives of This Handbook

Does the HIM department need continuous quality improvement?

Always a vital component of healthcare, health information management (HIM) is becoming an even more important component of reimbursement, accreditation, corporate compliance, and, of course, patient care. Indeed, few functions within a healthcare organization are not affected, at some level, by the information stored in patient medical records. For that reason, HIM departments cannot afford to let performance slip—or even stall. HIM staff must constantly seek opportunities for change that will improve the accuracy and timeliness of all HIM functions.

What if the department is running well?

CQI can make effective departments even better. For too long, HIM departments have viewed quality improvement as a *reactive* tool for addressing *visible* problems. But departments that have embraced truly effective CQI don't wait for problems to arise. They embrace a cycle of continuous change that prevents problems. They rely on CQI to help them refine departmental priorities, enhance performance, improve cash-flow, and, most importantly, increase the quality of patient care—even when department performance is, by all accounts, satisfactory.

How can this book help?

This book, *Continuous Quality Improvement for Health Information Management*, is a practical, how-to guide for HIM professionals who care about quality. Designed to help you tap the full potential of CQI, it introduces relevant concepts, terms, and tools. It demonstrates, through a series of in-depth case studies, how today's HIM departments are using CQI to address some of the most pressing issues in healthcare. And it outlines a step-by-step process for implementing a CQI program and making CQI principles part of your department's culture.

How is this book different?

No other book is specifically designed to apply CQI tools and techniques in an HIM context. *Continuous Quality Improvement for Health Information Management* is concise, easy to understand, and easy to use. It provides clear, relevant examples, and the book's CQI planner and inservice kit will make it easier to introduce key concepts to HIM staff and other audiences throughout your organization.

What does this book cover?

Chapter 2: CQI Basics

This chapter provides an overview of key principles and concepts. It profiles quality and management gurus whose thinking paved the way for today's CQI. Included here is a discussion of:

- W. Edwards Deming and his 14-point management strategy;
- Joseph M. Juran and the Quality Trilogy;
- Brian Joiner and the Joiner Triangle;
- Philip Crosby and his Four Quality Absolutes.

Chapter 3: Applying CQI to HIM

This chapter takes quality concepts that were initially developed for business and industry, and addresses them in the context of health information management. Specifically it applies Deming's "14 Points" to HIM, and it introduces 11 keys to implementing CQI effectively within an HIM department. This chapter also addresses the role that CQI can play in securing and protecting JCAHO accreditation.

Chapter 4: CQI Tools

This chapter introduces 15 tools that are an integral part of data-driven CQI. These tools can help you identify opportunities for improving existing processes, point you toward effective improvement initiatives, and support monitoring of those initiatives. Brief overviews of the tools are followed by more specific information on how and when to use each one, and by helpful illustrations.

Chapter 5: Case Studies

This chapter provides real-life examples of CQI in action. It takes a look at how your peers are addressing some of the most challenging issues in HIM, and it puts CQI theory in a practical light.

Chapter 6: CQI Planner

This chapter provides the step-by-step guidance you'll need to implement CQI in your department. It provides an 18-step, 18-month workplan and a timeline that will help you organize your department's shift to a CQI culture.

Chapter 7: CQI Inservice Kit

This chapter is designed to help you generate support for CQI throughout your department and organization. It includes tips on public speaking, and it provides a presentation outline and overheads for an inservice session that will introduce your staff to CQI. The sample overheads included in this chapter are yours to use as is, or as a guide for developing a customized session.

Appendix: Resource Guide

The resource guide in the book's appendix lists information on organizations, publications, and other materials that can further assist your efforts to build an effective CQI program.

Chapter 2:
CQI Basics

Chapter 2: CQI Basics

What is quality?

The term "quality" means different things to different people. To some, it implies adherence to a predetermined set of standards. To others, it means maintaining a high level of service and customer satisfaction. Whatever your definition, though, achieving and improving quality must be continuous activities within health information management (HIM).

In HIM, quality has many facets, and assessing quality depends on a number of indicators. Quality HIM service involves, for instance, the timely maintenance of accurate, complete chart documentation—including information on patient demographics, diagnoses, orders, procedures, and treatment outcomes. It entails precise and timely analysis and coding, responsive and responsible release of information, and timely reimbursement. And quality HIM service can also mean maintaining an accurate and complete master patient index, effectively routing records to physicians and others, accurately tracking the location of unfiled charts, and properly assembling records. There are, in short, a lot of factors that help determine the overall "quality" of service and performance in HIM and, of course, many opportunities for that quality to lapse.

What is continuous quality improvement?

Continuous quality improvement (CQI) is a data-driven process for improving performance that is fueled by an open-minded, thoughtful evaluation of opportunities for change. It involves looking proactively at an organization's functions, services, and products and asking, "How can we do better?" At its most basic level, CQI is a tool for responding to existing problems, but the ideal quality-management system uses CQI techniques to prevent problems or to uncover opportunities for improving an otherwise acceptable status quo.

The terms "continuous quality improvement" and "quality assurance" (QA) are often used interchangeably. However, they are different concepts. QA involves looking for problems retrospectively. It often assumes that some amount of error or imperfection is inevitable and, therefore, acceptable. CQI, on the other hand, involves ongoing, proactive assessment and the rejection of error or imperfection at any level.

Embracing CQI means welcoming an atmosphere that encourages change and seeks it out. It means accepting the notion that processes and products can always be improved through analysis, and that each error, defect, complaint, or inefficiency—no matter how small—represents an opportunity for improvement.

Many tools are available to facilitate CQI analysis (see Chapter 4, "CQI Tools"). They generate and organize concrete, statistical evidence that can help shape and support improvement initiatives. CQI tools are valuable resources for implementing analysis, communicating findings, charting the progress of initiatives, and projecting future directions for change.

Quality pioneers

Definitions for quality and approaches to CQI differ in subtle but significant ways, and the fundamental techniques and concepts underlying each approach to CQI are the same: Management must train employees to analyze processes, give them the authority to initiate change, and encourage them to use that authority. But each has its roots in the thinking of a few quality pioneers: W. Edwards Deming, Joseph M. Juran, Philip Crosby, and Brian Joiner.

W. Edwards Deming

Perhaps the most notable of the early quality pioneers is W. Edwards Deming, whose theories first gained influence in Japan during the 1950s. One of Japan's highest quality awards is the Deming Award, and his theories are now applied worldwide.

Deming outlines a 14-point approach to managing for maximum quality (see Figure 2.1). It forms the core of his philosophy, and it can serve as the basis for integrating CQI into the culture of nearly any organization. Chapter 3 places these 14 points in a context that's more specific to HIM.

Deming's approach often necessitates a dramatic shift in management styles, one that is designed to help make change-mindedness and CQI an integral part of an organization's culture. Deming calls for the elimination of management practices that discourage change and are not conducive to excellence. To this end, Deming identifies Seven Deadly Diseases (see Figure 2.2)—seven obstacles to change that exist, in some form, within most organizations. The first five "diseases" reflect general

Figure 2.1

Deming's 14 Points

1. Create constancy of purpose for improvement of product and service.
2. Adopt the new philosophy.
3. Cease dependence on mass inspection.
4. End the practice of awarding business on price tag alone.
5. Improve constantly and forever the system of production and service.
6. Institute training.
7. Institute leadership.
8. Drive out fear.
9. Break down barriers between staff areas.
10. Eliminate slogans, exhortations, and targets for the work force.
11. Eliminate numerical quotas.
12. Remove barriers to pride in workmanship.
13. Institute a vigorous program of education and retraining.
14. Take action to accomplish the transformation.

Figure 2.2

Deming's Seven Deadly Diseases

1. *Lack of constancy of purpose:* Any organization that does not have a defined purpose or long-range plan will most likely have insecure employees and dissatisfied customers.
2. *Emphasis on short-term profits:* When the only goal is to meet a budget or realize a projection, quality tends to suffer.
3. *Merit ratings or annual reviews:* Handled poorly, these can prompt destructive competition between workers, discouraging teamwork and damaging employee morale.
4. *Mobility of management:* Turnover or "job-hopping," particularly among management, interferes with the long-term plans of organizations and the career goals of employees.
5. *Running an organization "by the numbers":* Focusing solely on financial goals often means organizations are not attuned to the satisfaction levels of customers and employees.
6. *Excessive medical costs:* The high cost of medical care for employees tends to increase the cost of goods and services.
7. *Excessive costs of warranty:* These costs are often fueled by lawyers who work on a contingency fee.

tendencies that create and support a hierarchical culture and that can eventually prompt inconsistencies and inefficiencies. They are often fueled by an excessive emphasis on maximizing profitability, and they usually generate employee dissatisfaction. The last two "diseases" identify specific factors that can undermine customer satisfaction and exacerbate the effects of the first five.

Joseph M. Juran

Joseph M. Juran is another quality pioneer who is known for his work with Japanese industry. He sees three components as being key to any quality program:

- Goal setting—based on customers or competition;
- Infrastructure—revising the infrastructure to facilitate change; and
- Resources—focusing on training and measuring quality.[1]

Juran believes that organizations need to find a more universal approach to thinking about quality, "one which fits all functions, all levels, and all product lines."[2] To help them accomplish this, he developed his "Quality Trilogy," three basic quality-oriented processes: 1) quality planning, 2) quality control, and 3) quality improvement.

1. Quality planning, for Juran, is guided by the needs of internal and external customers. The key step in this stage of the trilogy involves identifying customers and their needs to better tailor products and services for them. Planning allows organizations to set quality-oriented goals, to develop products designed to facilitate quality service, and to establish processes that are driven primarily by an emphasis on quality and quality improvement.

2. The quality-control stage in Juran's trilogy entails establishing parameters to focus quality initiatives; organizations decide which functions and processes to target, which measurement tools and performance standards to apply, and, ultimately, which changes to propose. This stage, in short, generates mechanisms for change.

---

[1] Juran, Joseph. Quality Progress. "The Quality Trilogy" (Wilton, CT: Juran Institute, August 1986), p. 20.

[2] Ibid.

3. Juran's quality-improvement stage involves applying the mechanisms established during the quality-control stage to achieve the goals outlined during the quality-planning stage. It means reforming existing processes to emphasize quality and to improve performance across an organization. Juran's quality improvement focuses on organizing a project, identifying the problems to be tackled, proposing solutions, implementing those solutions, and assessing the results.

Each of these processes, argues Juran, is closely related to financial mechanisms that already exist within most organizations (see Figure 2.3), and no one process can be allowed to dominate the others.

Figure 2.3

Juran's Quality and Finance Parallels

Trilogy processes	Financial processes
1. Quality planning	Budgeting
2. Quality control	Cost control, expense control
3. Quality improvement	Cost reduction, profit improvement

Reproduced with permission from the copyright holder, Juran Institute, Inc., Wilton, CT 06897.

Philip Crosby

Philip Crosby, a third well-known quality consultant, has established four "quality absolutes" for improving the performance and service of organizations and individuals (see Figure 2.4). He insists that quality must be standards-based—that is, built around a set of clear, objective requirements rather than something as subjective as what "seems" good. He says that eliminating the root causes of problems is the first step to real improvement, and he insists that the ultimate goal must be zero defects. It's not enough, according to Crosby, to approach zero. Crosby also suggests that, when debating the cost of quality initiatives, organizations should consider the potential costs of not acting. Like Deming, Crosby emphasizes the importance of educating and empowering an entire organization, not just management or senior management.

Figure 2.4

Crosby's Quality Absolutes

1. Quality is defined as conformance to requirements, not "goodness."
2. The system for causing quality is prevention, not appraisal.
3. The performance standard must be zero defects, not "that's close enough."
4. The measurement of quality is the price of nonconformance, not indexes.

©The Creative Factory, Inc. Reprinted by permission of Philip Crosby Associates II, Inc.

Brian Joiner

Brian Joiner, a quality consultant and proponent of Deming's philosophies, believes that a culture of continuous quality improvement starts at the top of an organization and works its way downward. The Joiner method focuses on training top management to identify problems and opportunities for improvement, then training employees to assist in proposing and implementing solutions. The Joiner Triangle outlines Joiner's three-faceted approach (see Figure 2.5).

Figure 2.5

The Joiner Triangle

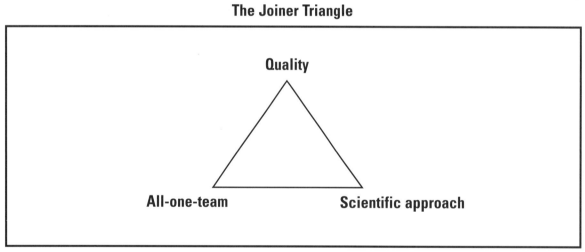

© 1988 Oriel, Inc. (formerly Joiner Associates). All rights reserved. Reprinted with permission.

Quality is at the top of the triangle because it is the ultimate goal of any CQI program. For Joiner, maximizing quality means focusing closely on customer needs and designing or redesigning products and services to meet them.

Improving quality, argues Joiner, should be a "scientific" process. He emphasizes using CQI tools and data to identify opportunities for improvement and to develop and measure proposed solutions. Processes are examined for flaws, and those flaws are addressed to create better, more productive systems.

In Joiner's model, teamwork is the key to CQI, and Joiner's emphasis on taking a team approach highlights the need for involvement in CQI at all levels of an organization. This approach requires creation of an environment, or organizational culture, that fosters change by allowing and encouraging all employees to contribute ideas. Joiner says an atmosphere of openness and acceptance breaks down barriers between and within departments, boosts morale, and increases commitment to the organization by creating a sense of ownership among all employees—all of which can lead to better performance.

Conclusion

True CQI is not an intermittent or retrospective process. It must be ongoing and proactive. It can be problem-oriented—that is, used to improve acknowledged flaws. But ideally, organizations use CQI to identify and seize opportunities for improvement—which may mean making something better simply because it is possible to do so.

Ultimately, the theories of the quality pioneers discussed above demand that organizations rethink traditional notions of top-down management and hierarchical structure. These theories suggest that management edicts do little to prompt significant change and improvement, that what organizations really need is top-down support for a CQI process that is driven and implemented by employees. Change-mindedness and improvement initiatives must be embraced and enacted at the bottom of an organization to have a real effect on quality. This means that management must be willing to hand the CQI reins to employees, to focus on channeling the creative energy and organizational know-how of those employees, and to commit to welcoming the input and to implementing the best ideas that result. It's not easy, but organizations that can make this shift will begin to establish an organizational culture that fosters true CQI and that embraces ongoing, quality-oriented change.

Chapter 3: Applying CQI to HIM

Chapter 3: Applying CQI to HIM

Applying Deming's 14 Points to health information management

W. Edwards Deming, a pioneering quality theorist, helped make CQI practices viable in the work place. His "14 Points" continue to provide a strong foundation for organizational improvement programs. This chapter is designed to help health information management professionals apply his thinking, and the theories of other quality pioneers. It begins by placing Deming's "14 Points" in an HIM context.

Point 1: Create constancy of purpose for improvement of product and service.

What are our products? What services does our department offer? Who are our customers? What are their needs? HIM departments that are dedicated to CQI ask these questions all the time. And as the answers to the last two evolve—that is, as customer demands shift—these departments find ways to ensure that their products and services keep pace. In short, Deming's first point requires that you know your customers (which for HIM departments can range from patients and medical staff, to the billing department and just about everything in between), and that you dedicate your department to providing the best customer service possible.

Point 2: Adopt the new philosophy.

Once you've established that constancy of purpose, your commitment to improving customer service cannot waver. CQI must, in other words, become an integrated part of your department's culture, and the organizational structure of the department may need to shift for that to happen. Creating self-directed work teams, and taking other steps to remove barriers that suffocate initiative and motivation, opens the door to real change; it empowers employees to examine work processes and department functions in the context of customer service, and it encourages them to propose ways of improving those processes and functions.

Point 3: Cease dependence on mass inspection.

Deming regularly emphasized the need for quality programs to be proactive, not reactive. "'Quality comes not from inspection,'" he has been quoted as saying, "'but from improvement in the process.'"[1] In an HIM context, this might mean

---

[1] *Walton, Mary. The Deming Management Method (New York: Putnam, 1986), p. 60.*

re-engineering processes to make them less prone to error and to reduce the need for retrospective quality reviews. For instance, evaluating the performance of transcriptionists, coders, and abstractors with the goal of identifying poor performance and correcting errors is not an efficient use of staff time, and it can create a confrontational atmosphere that's damaging to morale. CQI is designed to identify and eliminate the root causes of performance problems—or, better yet, to allow departments to seize opportunities for improvement before problems emerge. This emphasis on operating proactively eliminates a lot of "rework" and allows employees to focus on performing the tasks for which they were hired.

Point 4: End the practice of awarding business on price tag alone.

Businesses must be cost-conscious, but they must also recognize that the cheapest option is not always the best one. The cost of rework may negate initial savings. And, from the standpoint of customer satisfaction, the "cost" of a cheap job done poorly often exceeds that of a more costly job done well. Spending a bit more on behalf of customers or employees may increase satisfaction and quality to levels that generate real bottom-line rewards. Satisfied HIM employees, for instance, may be more productive, more efficient, and more accurate, which can have a direct effect on the speed and accuracy of billing. When making staffing-, vendor-, and other cost-related decisions, therefore, departments must carefully weigh pressures to limit spending against the legitimate needs of internal and external customers.

Point 5: Improve constantly and forever the system of production and service.

For CQI to work, every person in your department must accept that it involves continuous assessment and adjustment. HIM, like healthcare in general, is evolving. Changes made last month or last year may be obsolete today or tomorrow. Cultivating change-mindedness within your department can keep you on the cutting edge of quality, but doing so requires hard work, teamwork, and commitment from everyone—management and staff alike.

Point 6: Institute training.

Substandard training produces substandard employees who don't do quality work. And in healthcare, quality lapses can cost lives, as well as dollars. It's crucial, therefore, for departments to invest resources in training programs that allow staff to fulfill their potential and to live up to management expectations. Workers who are trained informally by colleagues, for instance, may learn the wrong methods or pick up bad habits. Poorly conceived training materials can be counterproductive, as well. Proper education and orientation, however, will help ensure that employees meet quality standards. They also give workers a solid knowledge base from which to propose changes and improvements.

Point 7: Institute leadership.

Leadership is the real job of management, and it involves far more than giving directives and punishing poor performance. A good leader assumes that employees are doing their best and provides tools—like additional training and an introduction to CQI—that will help them keep improving. This kind of guidance and support empowers and motivates employees. It generates a sense of commitment that's crucial to ensuring quality performance and customer service. Good leaders, in other words, know how to distribute power and responsibility in ways that encourage commitment, motivation, and resolve.

Point 8: Drive out fear.

Employees may hesitate to point out a problem or share an idea if they fear punishment or embarrassment, or if they sense that managers don't value their opinions. Consequently, problems fester because the people who could address them are not inclined to do so. Successful CQI programs seek to eliminate the sources of fear that are generally associated with the acknowledgment and identification of problems. Managers committed to CQI encourage employees to drive the improvement process by demonstrating a strong commitment to change-mindedness and by listening to and acting upon employee suggestions and concerns.

Point 9: Break down barriers between staff areas.

No hospital department or area of HIM is autonomous; each works directly or indirectly with many others. Because that's true of day-to-day work functions, it must also be true of CQI initiatives. Improvement efforts may not be effective unless they are embraced throughout your organization and department. CQI goals and procedures need to be consistent within and across departments. The importance of teamwork, communication, and commitment cannot be overstated.

Point 10: Eliminate slogans, exhortations, and targets for the work force.

Deming's tenth point is related to number seven (institute leadership) in that it involves relationships between management and staff. As noted previously, effective

CQI is generally driven by employees—the people who are closest to the processes under examination. But it should be sponsored and supported by management. Slogans, exhortations, and performance targets generally indicate limited employee input. Managers who rely on them are often dictating to employees, and they may appear unwilling to confront the real issues affecting performance and quality. Telling an under-staffed or poorly equipped HIM department to "work smarter, not harder," for instance, makes a manager seem unreasonable and out of touch; it's likely to create an us-versus-them mentality that actually discourages employees. Discussing issues honestly with employees and, more importantly, empowering employees to use CQI to do something about the problems, challenges, and opportunities that confront your department may foster the teamwork and commitment that are so crucial to improving quality and performance.

Point 11: Eliminate numerical quotas.

In general, quotas do not improve employee performance. Emphasis on transcribing a set number of lines, abstracting so many records, or coding a randomly chosen number of diagnoses rarely improves quality. In fact, rigid quotas may reduce quality and accuracy by prompting staff to rush complex tasks in an effort to meet an unreasonable or unrealistic standard. The focus should rest, instead, on providing the best possible service and quality—even if that means working more slowly. Replace quantitative standards with qualitative ones, and encourage employees to work efficiently but at a realistic pace; quality and productivity will improve as a result.

Point 12: Remove barriers to pride in workmanship.

HIM staff who are not properly trained, who work with faulty equipment, who feel they have little control over their workplace and their jobs, and who feel that they cannot discuss departmental issues with supervisors are less likely to take pride in a job well done. People are normally motivated to do the best job possible, but that motivation wanes if lack of training, poor equipment, or a dissatisfying work environment undermines them. A CQI program can help eliminate such barriers. Furthermore, encouraging development and implementation of an employee-driven CQI program can instill a sense of ownership that increases employee commitment to quality.

Point 13: Institute a vigorous program of education and retraining.

Education and continuous training are essential to any CQI program. They help demonstrate management's commitment to quality and change, and to the development of employee skills. A significant percentage of the HIM budget should, therefore, be devoted to training—both in CQI techniques, and to help employees hone other job-related skills. Initial training should cover information relevant to specific work assignments, and should be designed to help employees master CQI. Ongoing training initiatives should foster employee growth and development by addressing new job- and CQI-related concepts.

Point 14: Take action to accomplish the transformation.
Committing to the shift in management paradigms that makes CQI both possible and effective takes courage and determination. Managers must be willing to get the process started and then hand over control of it to their employees. Departments may need to commit time and resources to studying and adapting the theories of Deming and others. HIM staff must learn to embrace change and to accept responsibility for initiating it. It's not a simple process, but taking action to adopt a CQI program is likely to make your department more effective and your work more satisfying.

Eleven keys to implementing CQI in HIM

As discussed in Chapter 2, approaches to CQI can differ, but many of the basic principles are the same. To further assist HIM departments and professionals, we've developed "11 Keys" for planning and organizing an effective CQI program:

Key 1: Create quality-oriented goals.
HIM directors should establish quality-oriented goals for each department function—from chart assembly and abstraction to coding, records retrieval, and records retention. This involves working with staff to identify the key components of each function and the general expectations of the department and its relevant customers. Then all department employees should assist in developing performance standards—not numerical quotas, but rather qualitative guidelines that communicate expectations and provide a performance gauge (see Figure 3.1). The standards should pertain to specific job-related responsibilities and, where relevant, should address aspects of customer service, like friendliness and responsiveness. Post all performance standards where employees can read them, and be sure to address them during training and orientation.

Figure 3.1

Sample Performance Standards: Filing and Retrieval

Key components	Expectations	Performance guidelines

• Record filing
• Loose-document filing
• Record retrieval
• Tracking unfiled records
	• Records available or easily located on demand
	• Loose documents are filed properly and promptly
	• Records are never lost
		• Complete records and loose documents filed within 24 hours
		• Retrieval within:
		  - 30 minutes of clinical requests
		  - 24 hours of reimburse-ment-related requests
		  - seven days of legal requests

Key 2: Identify customers and their needs.

Identifying customers is an essential part of any CQI initiative; in fact, it's generally one of the first steps that CQI teams take (see the case studies in Chapter 5). Your department's customer list must include everyone who depends upon the information and services that you provide—including internal customers (e.g., doctors, nurses, billing-office staff, etc.) and external customers (patients, government agencies, vendors, etc.).

Once you've identified a customer, determine their specific needs (see Figure 3.2 for a sample customer profile)—by brainstorming, perhaps, or by surveying them (Chapter 4 addresses brainstorming, surveying, and other CQI tools). Then set goals and guidelines for meeting these needs (see Key 1). If you find that customers expect too much, negotiate new performance parameters and standards. A key part of improving customer service and quality involves communicating the limitations of your department and managing customer expectations.

Figure 3.2

Sample Customer Profile

Customer: finance department

Customer expectation: timely access (within 72 hours) to accurate information on patient diagnoses, procedure codes, admission and discharge dates, payer information, etc.

Key 3: Work CQI into training and job-evaluation programs.

HIM management should establish interactive training and job-evaluation programs for staff that address CQI techniques and that encourage employees to use those techniques. These programs should emphasize the department's commitment to quality and to CQI. They should also include a discussion of the department's performance standards. In fact, an extended session might be an ideal setting in which to develop the standards. To demonstrate management's commitment to training, evaluation, and CQI, consider holding these sessions off-site. This will allow employees to escape daily responsibilities and focus more closely on the session. Furthermore, willingness to "break the routine" demonstrates management's commitment and may help engage employees.

Key 4: Cultivate employee ownership.

If departments are going to hold employees responsible for poor performance, they must also give staff the ability to control and recommend improvements to the work processes that affect performance. In short, management must grant employees "ownership" of the functions for which they are responsible, including the CQI process. Granting employees legitimate authority can increase their commitment to quality and encourage the entrepreneurial spirit that's a crucial part of CQI. In addition, employees are more likely to embrace change initiatives that they had a hand in developing.

Key 5: Encourage teamwork.

Management needs constantly to emphasize that HIM is an integral part of a larger team—a team that is ultimately responsible for delivering quality patient care. HIM departments also must address barriers to teamwork that exist within HIM and between departments. The more staff see themselves as a key link in the overall chain of care, the more emphasis they will place on customer service, and the more likely they will be to engage in meaningful CQI.

Key 6: Implement a system for capturing suggestions.

No one knows a job better than the person who performs it. Likewise, no one can identify the strengths and weaknesses of a process better than the employees who function within it daily. That's why it's important to include staff in the CQI process (as opposed to issuing top-down edicts mandating change). Suggestion boxes and idea boards are simple mechanisms for encouraging and capturing employee input and for demonstrating management-level commitment to the CQI process. However, the ideas generated by such mechanisms must be acknowledged, evaluated, and implemented; otherwise employees will lose faith in the process.

Key 7: Establish a system for tracking and responding to complaints.

It's also important to create mechanisms that allow employees and customers to lodge complaints. Whereas your suggestion box or idea board is designed to capture change proposals, a complaint box or board allows the department to begin spotting opportunities for change. Customer surveys and hotlines are also excellent tools for capturing this kind of information. Creating such mechanisms may help employees and customers overcome the fear of raising negative issues in front of supervisors and colleagues. As with suggestions (see Key 6), though, it's not enough simply to collect complaint-related input; it's important to respond to complaints with meaningful reform initiatives.

Key 8: Monitor performance indicators.

For CQI to be truly continuous, departments must establish mechanisms that allow for ongoing monitoring of key performance indicators. Quality audits and monitoring reports (see Figure 3.3) are an effective way to gather such information. Audits can be retrospective (e.g., via chart reviews). However, that's a time-consuming process, and since retrospective evaluations take place after the fact, the information you gather may be slightly dated. Computer technology is making concurrent auditing and monitoring more feasible (see the case study in Chapter 5 entitled "CQI Averts Delinquent Records Crisis" for information on an organization that's using computerized bar-coding technology for performance monitoring).

Figure 3.3

Sample Quality-Monitoring Report
(Department Performance Indicators)

	Comparison figure or benchmark	month 1	month 2 → month 12	
Coding/Abstracting				
(total # records)				
% of coding errors (acceptable range __% to __%)				
% of abstracting errors (acceptable range __% to __%)				
% of records requiring re-abstracting/recoding (acceptable range __% to __%)				
% of records not coded or abstracted within _____ days of discharge				
Filing/Retrieving				
(total # records)				
% of records not pulled within				
_____ minutes of a clinical request				
_____ hours of a reimbursement request				
_____ days of a legal request				
_____ hours of a patient's request				
# records misplaced for > 30 days				
# orphaned (loose) documents that require filing				
Transcription				
#/% histories & physicals, operative reports transcribed within 24 hours				
#/% stat reports transcribed within 24 hours				
#/% errors in transcribed reports				
#/% blanks left in transcribed reports				
Release of Information				
(total # requests)				
#/% requests not responded to within: 24 or 48 hours, 1 week, 2 weeks, etc.				
#/% second requests				

Figure 3.3 (cont.)

Sample Quality-Monitoring Report

	Comparison figure or benchmark	month 1	month 2 → month 12	
Release of Information (cont.)				
#/% complaints regarding release of information				
#/% of compliments				
Customer Service				
#/% complaints from:				
- patients				
- physicians				
- third parties				
#/% compliments from:				
- patients				
- physicians				
- third parties				
Customer-satisfaction index (based on formal or informal surveys) (acceptable range is ___ to ___)				
Management				
Average # sick days for all employees (acceptable range __ to __)				
% overtime/regular hours (acceptable range __% to __%) (standard is < 2%)				
Employee turnover				
% resigned				
% fired				
% hired				
% performance appraisals done on time (acceptable range __% to __%)				

Other Indicators

What indicators in your department provide meaningful information on the quality of services provided?_____

Key 9: Monitor the vital signs of quality efforts.

Once your department has embraced CQI, it's important to monitor employee enthusiasm for the process. Maintaining momentum can be difficult, and one key challenge for management is finding ways to keep employees interested. Support for the process, and commitment to the goal of integrating CQI into the daily culture of the department, must trickle down from the senior levels of an organization.

Key 10: Recognize employee quality efforts.

Don't let employees think that you take their efforts and their input for granted. Recognizing their ideas and contributions is a key way for management to demonstrate support for CQI without taking control of the process away from the staff. Small rewards—even a simple "thank you"—can go a long way toward generating broad support for CQI.

Key 11: Develop improvement teams.

While you want all employees to contribute ideas for change and improvements, it often makes sense to establish a CQI team to oversee the formal assessment of specific functions. The camaraderie and sense of shared purpose that exists within the group may help them work more effectively. Teams also help make CQI an interdisciplinary process by providing a vehicle for bringing together people from different parts of the organization. In addition, management's willingness to allocate time and resources to a team can be a powerful demonstration of an organization's commitment to CQI.

CQI and JCAHO accreditation

The JCAHO has long recognized that CQI can have a positive impact on the quality of patient care in hospitals and other healthcare organizations. For that reason, the JCAHO's performance improvement (PI) standards require facilities to have formalized, systematic mechanisms in place for measuring and assessing data on patient care, treatment outcomes, and other key functions, and for launching improvement initiatives based on their findings. The JCAHO also requires that performance-improvement efforts be collaborative and interdisciplinary.

CQI is also an effective means for ensuring compliance with other JCAHO standards, including some that govern HIM processes. CQI tools and techniques allow organizations to evaluate relevant processes, to determine whether those processes are likely to meet the expectations of JCAHO surveyors, and, if they are not, to fashion improvements that make those processes compliant.

Since the JCAHO reorganized its accreditation manuals in 1994, HIM departments have had to comply with standards in several chapters, but the largest concentration of relevant standards is in the *Management of Information* (IM) section. To use hospital standards as an example, the most notable for HIM departments are, perhaps, those requiring organizations 1) to monitor and report treatment- and outcome-related data, and 2) to include information in medical records that identifies patients, supports diagnoses, justifies treatment decisions and orders, tracks the results of treatment, and ensures continuity of care if multiple providers see or treat a patient. Among other things, JCAHO standards also require medical records to document specific procedures—like operations and administration of anesthesia. The standards demand that facilities protect the security and confidentiality of patient information—including, of course, anything contained in the medical record. And they mandate that organizations collect and transmit data to authorized audiences in a timely and accurate manner. These are just a few of the HIM-related processes that CQI teams can monitor and analyze, and for which they can generate data-driven improvement initiatives.

The HIM department should lead CQI assessments of processes related to documentation in medical records (see Figure 3.4 for a step-by-step guide to staging a documentation-improvement initiative). And since the medical record is often an integral source of data for other collection vehicles (registries, for instance), the department should consider leading—and it should definitely participate in—CQI inquiries that target those vehicles (see the case study in Chapter 5 entitled "Making the Most of Databases and Registries" for an example of one such initiative).

Articles in recent years have criticized some approaches to CQI for focusing more on process than outcomes. When one takes into account the statistical intricacies involved in formal CQI analysis, or when one considers the bureaucracies often associated with federal regulation and with accreditation, it is possible to see how teams might be distracted by process—how they might wind up "going through the motions" in an effort, for instance, to satisfy JCAHO requirements. As valuable as CQI can be for securing and preserving organizational accreditation status, though, it's important never to lose sight of the ultimate goal: improving patient care. Organizations must avoid getting so preoccupied with monitoring and assessment activities that actual improvement falls by the wayside.

Figure 3.4

Assessing Records Documentation

To determine if the documentation in your medical records will pass muster with JCAHO standards, conduct a documentation-improvement project. Here's how:

1. Assemble an interdisciplinary task force to plan and conduct a review of chart documentation. Include representatives from the medical staff, HIM, nursing, finance, and other departments whose processes depend upon accurate, timely documentation.
2. Generate baseline data by reviewing a representative sampling of medical records (see Chapter 4 for an overview of tools that can help). Review at least 100 records to see how well the documentation meets the JCAHO's requirements.
3. List and prioritize the problems that your team discovers (cause-and-effect diagrams and decision matrices—see Chapter 4—are particularly useful for prioritizing).
4. Use quality improvement tools (see Chapter 4) to determine the underlying causes of problems and to shape improvement proposals.
5. Implement improvements and collect data to help you assess their effectiveness.
6. Make adjustments to improvement proposals that aren't working as effectively as planned. Take steps to institutionalize revised processes that are working.
7. Conduct quarterly reviews of medical records to ensure the continued compliance of documentation, or to catch additional quality lapses.

Chapter 4:
CQI Tools

Chapter 4: CQI Tools

Introduction

CQI involves making scientifically generated improvement proposals—initiatives that are based on data, not on instinct or "guesstimates." In this chapter, we describe 15 tools for collecting, analyzing, and/or displaying data. While other, more sophisticated, tools and analysis techniques exist, those highlighted here are the most common and the easiest to use.

Our descriptions include a basic overview of the tool in question. Then there is more specific information—for instance, on how and when to apply the tool. We also provide hints that are designed to help you use each tool as effectively as possible.

Later chapters supplement the information included here. The case studies in Chapter 5 show how organizations have put some of these tools to work. The sample presentation slides in Chapter 7 ("CQI Inservice Kit") include information on the tools that will add depth to your efforts to educate staff about CQI.

Bar graph

Overview

A bar graph allows you to compare the relative size of different data sets or of the component parts of one data set. They allow you to track trends and/or draw comparisons between items—comparisons that may help you set priorities.

When to use a bar graph

Use a bar graph when you want to understand how different sets of data compare with each other. For example, if you wanted to make a month-to-month comparison of the number of coding errors committed by each coder on your staff, a bar graph would allow you to organize raw data so that assessment could be made quickly and easily.

Different types of bar graph
Simple bar graph

A simple bar graph (see Figure 4.1) is useful when you are measuring one set of data that cannot be (or does not need to be) stratified or broken into sub-categories.

Figure 4.1

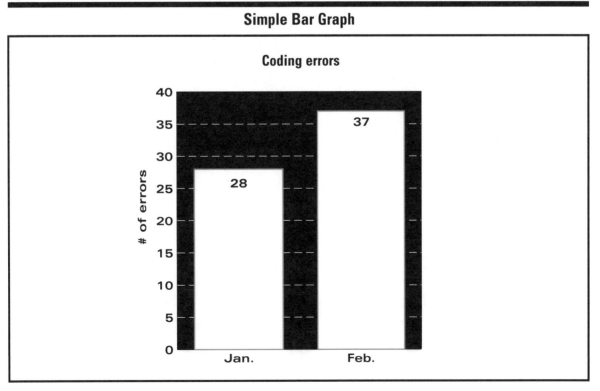

Simple Bar Graph

Coding errors

Clustered bar graph

If the totals displayed in a simple bar graph can be divided into subtotals, you might choose to display the data using a clustered bar graph. In Figure 4.2a, for instance, each narrow bar in the three-bar clusters displays a subtotal of the data displayed in Figure 4.1. Add the amounts displayed in three subtotal bars for each cluster, and they equal the "total" amount represented in the simple bar graph. Stack the narrow bars, and they would reach to the same height as the single bar in Figure 4.1. Clustered bar graphs are particularly useful if you want a format that emphasizes the relative impact of component subtotals on an overall total.

Figure 4.2a

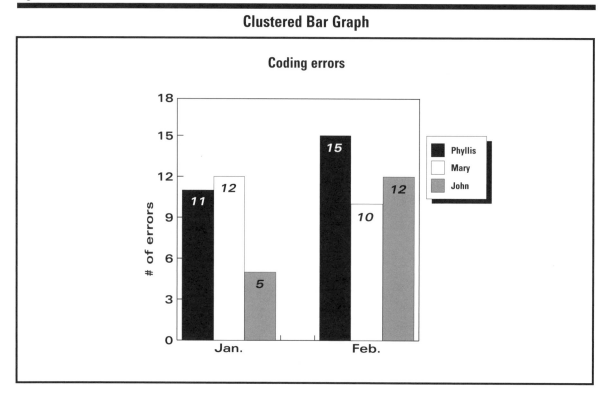

Stratified bar graph

Like a clustered bar graph, the stratified bar graph allows you to display subtotals. In this instance, however, a single bar representing the overall total is divided horizontally into proportional segments that represent each relevant subtotal (see Figure 4.2b). Whereas the clustered-bar-graph format subtly shifts the emphasis away from the grand total and onto the subtotal amounts, stratified bar graphs allow you to display subtotals while continuing to stress the grand total.

Figure 4.2b

Stratified Bar Graph

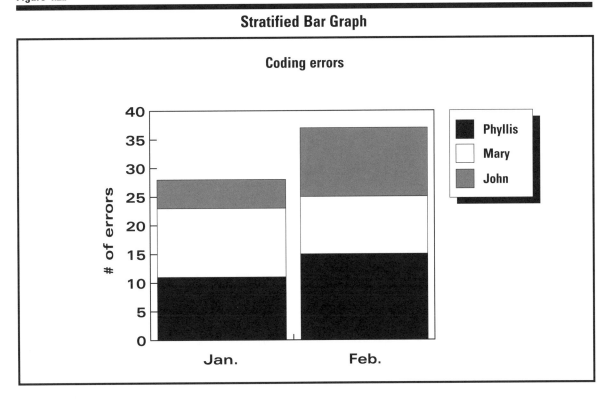

Coding errors

Putting bar graphs to work

Step 1

Collect raw data relevant to the process that you wish to evaluate.

Step 2

Choose which bar-graph format best suits your purposes in displaying the raw data.

Step 3

Decide how many bars you will need. This will determine the length of your horizontal x-axis.

Step 4

Identify the largest value among the data sets you collected. This will determine the scale for your vertical y-axis (the highest value on your scale should exceed the highest value in your data sets to ensure that your bars aren't taller than your graph).

Step 5

Draw bars that reach up to the level on the y-axis that corresponds with the total value that you measured for that item.

Hints

- The tallest bar on your graph will tend to be perceived as the most important or significant. If you want to call attention to a different bar, consider shading that other bar differently from the others so it stands out.
- Bar graphs are not well suited for displaying patterns in data over time. Consider using a run chart if you want to show how a process changes and fluctuates over a certain period of time.

Brainstorming

Overview

Brainstorming is a CQI tool used to generate as many ideas as possible on a particular subject. Either groups or individuals can brainstorm. Sessions should be spontaneous and unstructured, and, to encourage creativity and to keep input flowing freely, all ideas should be recorded without comment or judgment. There are no bad ideas and no good ideas when you brainstorm; there are only ideas.

When to use brainstorming

Use brainstorming when you want to encourage creativity and a free flow of ideas. It's a great way to get new CQI processes started or to revive stalled initiatives.

How to use brainstorming

Eliminate distractions and try to create an atmosphere that's designed to inspire participants and release creativity. Brainstorming sessions should be fun, lively, and not particularly long (an hour or less). The session facilitator should introduce the topic and the session's objectives, then urge people to say anything that comes to mind. As the session progresses, the facilitator should ask questions and introduce sub-topics that will help maintain the group's momentum.

Who uses brainstorming

Group sessions should include people with direct knowledge of the subject at hand. However, it's often also useful to involve people who know little or nothing at all about that subject; they're often the people who will ask simple questions or make off-beat suggestions that propel the whole group in especially creative directions. Group sessions need to be large enough to generate a lot of ideas, but small enough to be manageable and ensure that everyone gets involved. Six to 12 people is generally a good size.

Putting brainstorming to work

Step 1

- Choose your subject.
- Select the people who will participate in the brainstorming session and notify them of the time and place.

- Secure a meeting room and supplies: chalkboard, flip chart, wall chart, and so on.
- Draw up a list of leading questions that will help get the session started or keep it moving.

Step 2

- Convene the brainstorming session. Describe its goals and set guidelines (e.g., no bad ideas, no judgments or critiques, etc.). Be clear that everyone should participate and that one person should not rule the entire session.

Step 3

- When the group has been briefed, ask a question or two to get them started.
- Write down every response on the chalkboard or flip chart. (You may want to have another person help you do this, but it should not be someone who is also expected to brainstorm.)
- Make sure that every person has a turn, and encourage shy people to speak up. If thoughts wane on one topic or question, bring up a new one to keep the session going.
- As facilitator, you should avoid judging ideas and remind others not to do so, too. Even positive responses ("That's a great idea!") can stifle creativity.
- Set a time limit for the discussion and stick to it. Don't worry about stopping early if the group seems to be losing momentum.

Step 4

- Ten or fifteen minutes before the session breaks up, glance through your goals and objectives for the session. If something hasn't been covered, point the team in that direction.
- Toward the end of the session, it may also be useful to begin clustering similar ideas to identify themes and patterns that might prompt additional thinking in key areas.

Step 5

- Thank members for their participation in the brainstorming session and tell them how you plan to use the ideas they've generated.

Hints

- As facilitator, carefully develop your leading questions to cover all aspects of the subject in question.

- Brainstorming individually before the group session will help you focus on the subject and will make the brainstorming process easier to explain to others.
- Think of brainstorming ideas as "rough draft" improvement initiatives. You will probably need to evaluate and refine the ideas before implementing the most promising ones. Other CQI tools, such as flow charts, cause-and-effect diagrams, and pareto charts, can help.
- Capitalize on the enthusiasm that successful brainstorming sessions can generate. As you're shaping rough ideas into feasible improvement initiatives, keep the people from the brainstorming session, who are not on your CQI team, informed of your progress. They may offer additional input that's helpful.

Cause-and-effect diagram

Overview

Cause-and-effect diagrams are especially useful for organizing and focusing lists of possible causes to identify "root causes" and to generate a clear and manageable list of next actions. It is sometimes called a "fishbone diagram" because of its shape (see Figure 4.3). It has also been called the Ishikawa diagram, after the man who refined its use.

Figure 4.3

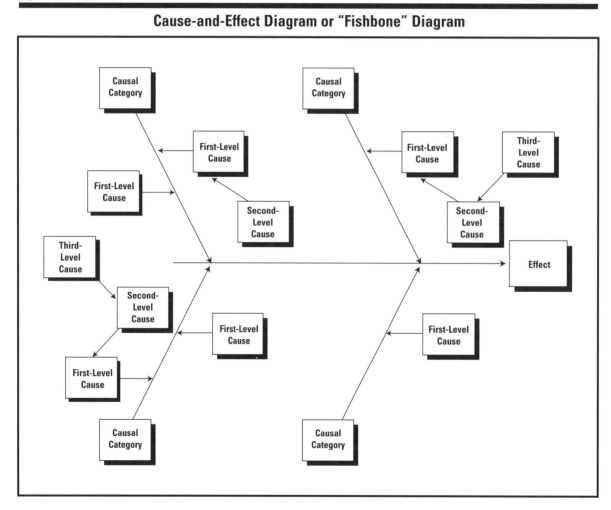

When to use a cause-and-effect diagram

Use the cause-and-effect diagram to isolate root causes for an effect, outcome, or problem.

How to use a cause-and-effect diagram

Begin with the "effect" and gradually work backward through layers of factors and causes until you've identified the most fundamental causes leading to that effect. Addressing these "root causes" will be the best way to alter the effect under examination.

Putting cause-and-effect diagrams to work

Step 1

Identify the problem or effect you want to address. Set up a brainstorming session to identify the root causes that produce that effect.

Step 2

Write a brief description of the "effect" in a box at the right side of the page and draw a line extending from it to the left (see Figure 4.4a). Think of the effect box as the "head" of your diagram and the line as the "spine."

Figure 4.4a

Diagram Head and Spine

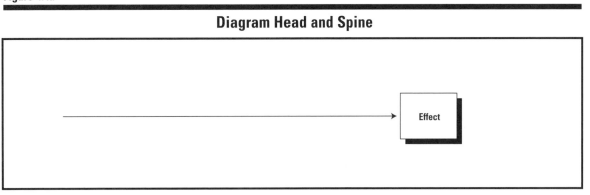

Effect

Step 3

Identify broadest possible factors or causes that are involved in producing the effect under examination (e.g., human actions, equipment, policies, etc.) and attach them to the diagram like ribs extending off a spine (see Figure 4.4b). Generally, these causal categories are too broad and ambiguous to be addressed effectively.

Step 4

Consider each "rib" separately; ask the group to brainstorm answers to the question, "Why or how does this contribute to the effect under examination?" The answers that

Figure 4.4b

Causal-Category Ribs

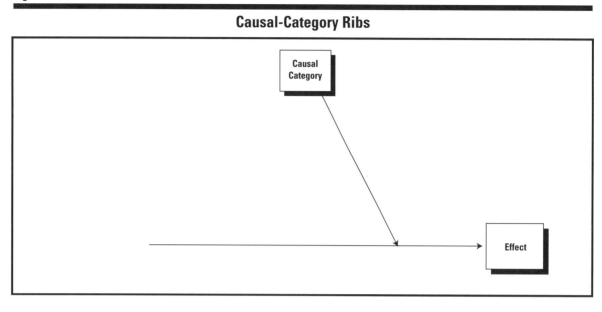

you generate are "first-level causes," and should be attached to the appropriate rib (see Figure 4.4c). These causes will be narrower, but may not yet be narrow enough to produce clear action steps or manageable improvement initiatives.

Figure 4.4c

First-Level Causes

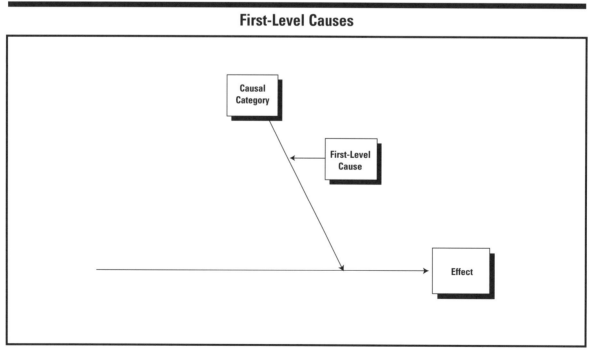

Step 5

If not, ask the same question about each first-level cause to generate second-level causes; from second-level causes, brainstorm third-level causes; and so on (see Figure 4.4d). Continue until you cannot focus the causes any further, or until the causes have become narrow enough that you can identify manageable action steps for addressing them. These are the root causes of the problem or effect in question.

Figure 4.4d

Additional Causal Levels

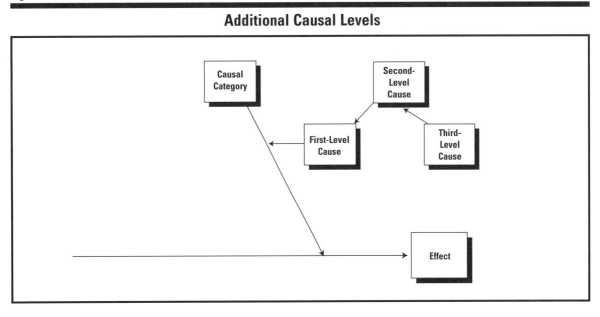

Step 6

Establish mechanisms for collecting data to verify that these root causes are, in fact, to blame for the problem or effect in question. This will help confirm the cause-and-effect analysis and help your team generate data-driven improvement proposals.

Hints

- The root causes identified by a cause-and-effect diagram represent "best guesses"—hypotheses that must be proven "scientifically" through the application of data-driven analysis.
- Be thorough in your search for root causes. The more layers you peel away in your search for root causes, the easier it will be to develop improvement initiatives that have far-reaching effects.
- Make sure that your team reaches consensus at each stage of cause-and-effect analysis before moving on to the next stage.

Check sheet

Overview

A check sheet is a grid that allows CQI teams to determine how often an event occurs. It will not identify the causes of that occurrence, but it can help teams prioritize action steps by revealing which events or problems occur with greatest frequency. A check sheet also identifies important patterns of occurrence. Check sheets often generate the raw data that is used to create pareto charts, histograms, run charts, and other tools that display data graphically.

When to use a check sheet

Use a check sheet any time you need to collect and classify raw data that has to do with the frequency of an event. For instance, a check sheet would be useful for tracking the number of delinquent records coming into your department each month, or for categorizing total delinquencies by doctor.

Putting a check sheet to work

Step 1

Identify the process you want to analyze and determine what data you will need to complete that analysis.

Step 2

Assign someone reliable to monitor the process in question and collect all relevant data. This person needs to be conscientious and detail-oriented. They must note each and every relevant occurrence, otherwise the data they collect will not be reliable.

Step 3

Choose categories for data collection (e.g., number of delinquent records per month, number of coding errors per shift, etc.).

Step 4

Create a check sheet grid. List the occurrences you want to tally down the left-hand column and put "tally categories" along the top (see Figure 4.5). You can then record individual event occurrences or occurrence totals in the appropriate box in the check-sheet grid.

Step 5

Begin collecting data, noting each occurrence of interest in the appropriate box (see Figure 4.6).

Figure 4.5

Check Sheet: Occurrence Totals

Major causes of incomplete records							
Causes	**Frequency over six months**						
Incomplete or missing:	**Jan**	**Feb**	**March**	**April**	**May**	**June**	**Total**
1. Histories & physicals	70	85	65	75	80	90	465
2. Attestations	140	150	135	145	160	170	900
3. Discharge summaries	125	130	140	135	130	130	790
4. Operative reports	60	80	95	90	120	100	545
5. Consultant reports	25	40	35	45	60	80	285
6. Signatures	150	165	170	155	170	200	1010
7. Other	80	50	70	35	40	70	345
Monthly Total	**650**	**700**	**710**	**680**	**760**	**840**	—

Figure 4.6

Check Sheet: Individual Occurrences

Analysis errors

Analysts / Day	Mon	Tue	Wed	Thu	Fri	Weekly Total (Individuals)
Polly	✓✓✓		✓✓			5
Joe		✓				1
Sue	✓			✓✓		3
Daily Total (Dept.)	4	1	2	2	0	9

Step 6

Once the data-collection process is complete, total each column and row.

Hints

- To better identify patterns or trends in the data you collect, use the raw data on your check sheet to generate a pareto chart, a histogram, a run chart, or some other tool that displays information graphically.
- Check sheets can be effective tools for continuous monitoring of key functions and performance indicators.
- Define data-collection categories as specifically as possible to ensure that collection efforts are consistent and data are reliable.

Decision matrix

Overview

A decision matrix is a grid that helps CQI teams objectively prioritize options. Those options are listed down the left-hand column, while criteria for evaluating them are noted along the top of the grid (see Figure 4.7). The team then scores each alternative, based on how well it fulfills the requirements of each criterion. The choice getting the highest total score is the top priority. Criteria can also be weighted so that more important ones have a greater impact on the total score (see Figure 4.8, and refer to the profile of Harris Methodist Hospital in Chapter 5, "Case Studies").

Figure 4.7

Decision Matrix

Possible action steps for increasing transcription turnaround time

Rating system: 1=Unimportant   2=Important   3=Very Important

Alternatives	Criteria			Total	Rank
	Cost-Effective	Time to Implement	Acceptability		
Upgrade equipment	*1*	*1*	*2*	*4*	*4*
Use outside services	*2*	*2*	*1*	*5*	*3*
Develop incentives for transcriptionists	*3*	*1*	*3*	*7*	*2*
Hire a clerk to file, look up numbers, etc.	*2*	*2*	*3*	*7*	*2*
Hire two more transcriptionists	*2*	*2*	*3*	*7*	*2*
Stop typing non-clinical reports	*3*	*3*	*3*	*9*	*1*

When to use a decision matrix

Decision matrices are helpful for performing "third-order" rankings of ideas and proposals. Brainstorming, for instance, identifies first-order CQI options (i.e., a list of ideas that have not been evaluated). Ideas that aren't feasible are then eliminated,

Figure 4.8

Decision Matrix with Weighted Criteria

		Quality Impact weight: 4	Cost Effectiveness weight: 5	Ease of Implementation weight: 5	Ability to Pilot weight: 5	Weighted-Score Total*	Rank
OPPORTUNITY AREAS	Fewer Reviews	2 / 8	3 / 15	2 / 10	3 / 15	48	3
	Share Information	1 / 4	3 / 15	1 / 5	2 / 10	34	5
	Idle Moments	1 / 4	3 / 15	2 / 10	3 / 15	44	4
	Data Integrity	3 / 12	3 / 15	2 / 10	3 / 15	52	2
	Opportunistic Collection	2 / 8	3 / 15	3 / 15	3 / 15	53	1
	Strategic Collection	3 / 12	3 / 15	2 / 10	3 / 15	52	2

Scoring	Weighting
How well does this opportunity area meet the goal of this criterion?	How important is this criterion relative to the others?
1 = poorly 2 = adequately 3 = well	3 = unimportant 4 = important 5 = very important
note scores to the left of the diagonals dividing the score boxes	*weighted score = score multiplied by criterion weight*

creating a list of "second-order" alternatives (i.e., viable options). A third-order ranking prioritizes those viable ideas.

How to use a decision matrix

Once the CQI team has generated a list of action items, improvement proposals, etc., have members establish criteria for evaluating each item on the list. This process may require discussion, negotiation, and compromise. Have each team member fill in the matrix separately, then combine their totals on a master matrix.

Putting decision matrices to work

Step 1

- Explain that decision-matrix analysis is designed to help make prioritizing as objective and scientific a process as possible.
- Suggest some criteria for evaluating the team's options, and ask team members to suggest others. You may want to hold a mini-brainstorming session (see page 47) to expand quickly your list of possible criteria.

Step 2

- Discuss each possible criterion and eliminate those that are least relevant.
- Weight the remaining criteria, if one or more are particularly crucial, and decide on a rating system with which to score your criteria. For example:
  - 1 = alternative fulfills few, if any, criterion requirements
  - 2 = alternative fulfills some criterion requirements
  - 3 = alternative fulfills most criterion requirements
  - 4 = alternative fulfills all criterion requirements

Step 3

- Give each participant a blank copy of the matrix (with alternatives down the left-hand side and criteria along the top) and have them score each alternative.
- Total the individualized scores on a master matrix.
- Assign top priority to the alternative that receives the highest total score on the master matrix. In Figure 4.7 (see page 57), for instance, the alternative "stop typing non-clinical reports" ranked highest, with a total score of 9 points. Three options are tied as the number two priority. To break the tie, team members could re-evaluate those three options on a separate matrix.

Step 4

- Take action, beginning with the top-priority option.

Hints

- CQI teams don't need to use decision matrices every time they're confronted with a list of options. Use them either when the number of possible options seems unmanageable or when time is limited and it's important to focus on a few key alternatives.
- When determining the criteria that the team will use to evaluate all options, identify as many possible criteria as you can before beginning to evaluate them. Trying to evaluate as you go along will bog the process down and discourage input.
- Don't worry about breaking ties unless they create a situation in which you'll still be forced to address too many options.
- When choosing criteria with which to rate alternatives, refer back to the overall goals of the CQI process. If, for instance, cost overruns are a problem in the department, you may want "cost-effectiveness" and/or "long-term impact on costs" to be heavily weighted.

Flow chart

Overview

Flow charts provide a graphical depiction of the sequence of steps needed to complete a process (see Figure 4.9). Using a standard set of symbols (see Figure 4.10), they indicate stopping and starting points, required actions, decision-making points, waiting periods, and needed documentation.

Figure 4.9

Flow Chart

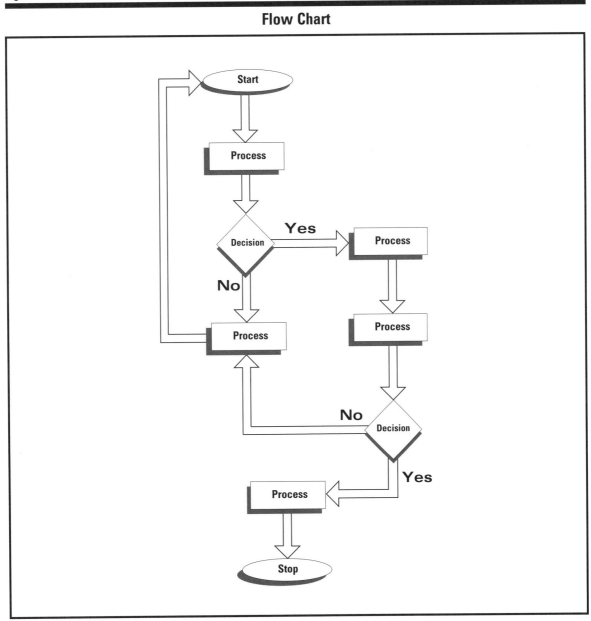

Figure 4.10

Flow Chart Symbols

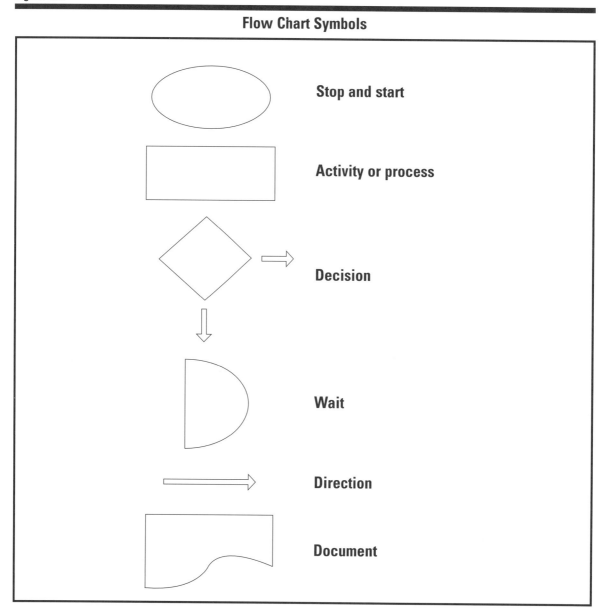

Stop and start

Activity or process

Decision

Wait

Direction

Document

When to use a flow chart

Use a flow chart any time you need to understand how an existing process affects the quality of the outcome that process is meant to generate. If, for instance, your department has a problem with delinquent records, a flow chart might reveal unnecessary delays and redundant steps in the records-completion process that contribute to delinquencies. Flow charts can also improve the use of other CQI tools—like surveys and brainstorming—because they identify each person who is involved in a process and could provide input.

How to use a flow chart

You can apply flow-chart analysis to any process, but it's crucial that you get the input of everyone who is involved in that process. Consider asking the people in your department who file loose reports, for example, to flow chart the steps that are involved in that process. Variations in their charts might reveal inefficiencies or a counterproductive lack of standardization.

Putting flow charts to work

Step 1

Identify the process that you want to analyze and begin a list of the steps involved in completing it.

Step 2

Show your list to others who are involved in the process and ask them to fill in any gaps. Be prepared to ask them specific questions in order to elicit as much detail about the process as possible.

Step 3

Organize your list of steps from start to finish.

Step 4

Use flow chart symbols (see Figure 4.10, page 62) to diagram the process.

Step 5

Connect all circles, boxes, and diamonds with arrows to indicate flow or direction. Be sure to explore all possible responses to a decision diamond (see Figure 4.11).

Step 6

Have others involved in the process evaluate your chart to check its accuracy and to help you locate possible inefficiencies in the process under examination.

Step 7

Where appropriate, propose changes that will streamline and/or improve the process.

Hints

- In order to create a flow chart that is both detailed and manageable, you may need to divide complex processes into their component sub-processes. Note, for instance, how the CQI team at Fairview Clinics (see Chapter 5, "Case Studies") separates the documentation and posting process into a number of sub-processes.

- It may be helpful to create master flow charts of the major functions in your department. This will facilitate future analysis. But be sure to update those master charts as department procedures evolve.
- Master flow charts can be useful training devices. They'll show new employees what their responsibilities are and give them something to refer to for reminders while they're on the job.
- Before you flow chart an actual process, it might be useful, in some instances, to diagram what you consider to be the ideal approach. Comparing the actual chart with the diagram of the "ideal" will help you identify improvement opportunities.

Figure 4.11

Decision Diamond

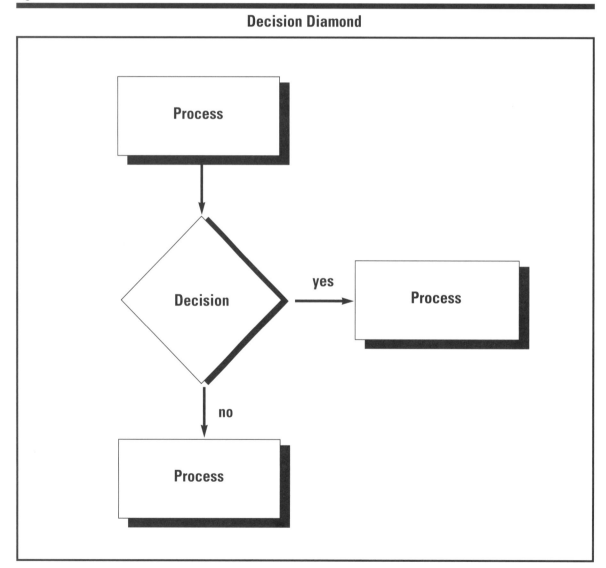

Histogram

Overview

A histogram is a form of bar graph that is useful for comparing patterns of occurrence over time—that is, it displays the frequency with which comparable events occur, and it illustrates variations in their occurrence. For instance, an HIM department might employ a histogram to chart trends in response-time to physicians' record requests (see Figure 4.12).

Figure 4.12

Histogram

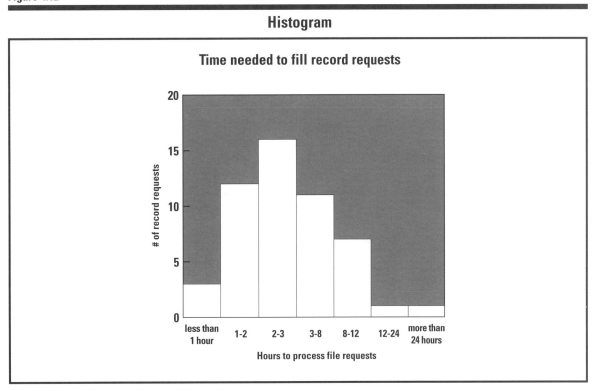

An analysis of Figure 4.12 indicates that most record requests are filled in three hours or less; however, it takes well over three hours to fill quite a few of them. If organizational policy requires that all record requests from physicians be filled in less than three hours, this histogram indicates slightly subpar performance. Note: Histograms generally measure frequency of occurrence on the vertical y-axis; they chart time (or the other significant variable being measured) along the horizontal x-axis.

When to use a histogram

Use a histogram to analyze trends and to identify variations in process completion. The process or action under examination should occur a minimum of 25 times over the period studied; histograms displaying fewer occurrences aren't generally very useful.

How to read a histogram

Histograms are useful, in part, because the shape or pattern formed by the array of bars can, at a glance, provide important information about the process under examination. For instance:

- A cluster of bars that peaks in the middle and has a narrow base suggests there is little performance variation in the process under examination (see Figure 4.13a).
- A cluster that peaks in the middle but has a wide base indicates a lot of performance variation (see Figure 4.13b).

Figure 4.13a

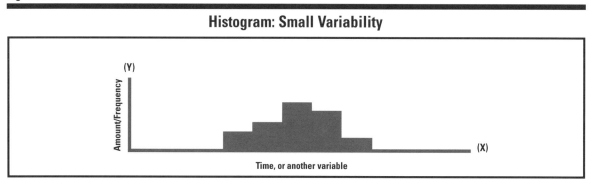

Histogram: Small Variability

Figure 4.13b

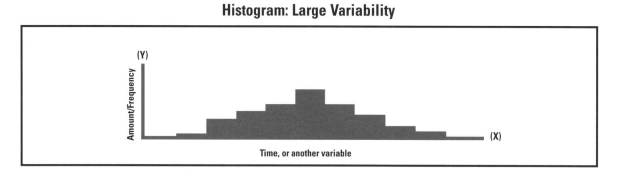

Histogram: Large Variability

- Histograms that peak on the left or right are known as skewed histograms; they indicate that something bizarre or unexpected happens occasionally during completion of the process (see Figure 4.13c).
- A histogram with two peaks indicates consideration of two incompatible data sets that should be reorganized in separate histograms (see Figure 4.13d).

Figure 4.13c

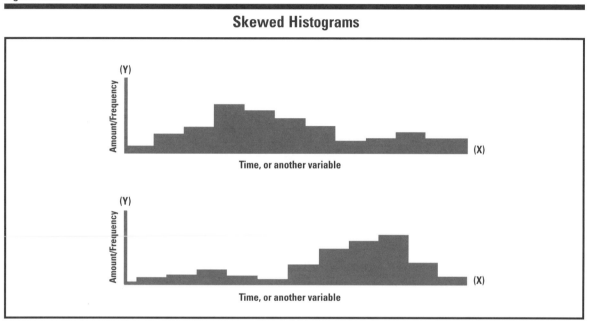

Skewed Histograms

Figure 4.13d

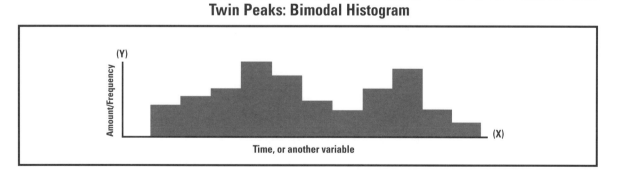

Twin Peaks: Bimodal Histogram

The first example above is sometimes called a "normal histogram"; it indicates that a process is, for the most part, proceeding as designed. The other examples indicate processes that probably need to be improved (provided the data that produced the histogram is accurate).

Putting a histogram to work

Step 1

Gather the raw data you will use to plot the histogram.

Step 2

Figure the range of your raw data by calculating the difference between the largest and smallest data points.

Step 3

Determine how many bars you'll use in your histogram by calculating the square root of the total number of data points collected.

Step 4

Determine the interval for each bar (the range of x-axis data that each bar will cover) by dividing the overall range by the number of bars. For a histogram with five bars and a data-point range of 50, for example, the interval for each bar would be 10 data points.

Step 5

Use a check sheet (see page 54) to group your raw data by intervals (see Figure 4.14a).

Step 6

Create your histogram. The total number of data points per interval determines the height of the bar for that class interval (see Figure 4.14b).

Step 7

Analyze the shape of the histogram and attempt to account for large variations, skews, or twin peaks.

Hint

- Abnormally shaped histograms could indicate defective processes. However, they might also indicate that your calculations or collection efforts were flawed. Always recalculate abnormal histograms before you begin exploring opportunities for changing the process under examination.

Figure 4.14a

Data for Histogram

Retrieval Times (raw)

35	28	50	38
42	15	43	42
28	3	45	25
35	10	20	8
30	20	22	11
32	25	36	19
11	55	23	15
9	46	28	30
6	78	7	60
53	45	19	3
27	28	30	50
18	16	26	36

Retrieval Times (arrayed)

3 3 6 7 8 9 10 10 11 13 15 16 17 18 19 19 20
20 22 23 25 25 26 27 28 28 28 28 29 29 30 30
30 32 35 35 35 36 36 38 42 42 43 45 45 46 47
50 50 53 55 55 60 78

Retrieval Time	Retrievals (per day)							
	Mon	Tues	Wed	Thur	Fri	Sat	Sun	Total
1-15 minutes	⦸⦸	‖		‖				11
16-30 minutes	‖‖	⦸	⦸‖	‖‖	‖‖			22
31-45 minutes	‖	‖‖		‖		‖		12
46-60 minutes						‖‖	⦸	8
over 60 minutes								1

Figure 4.14b

Histogram

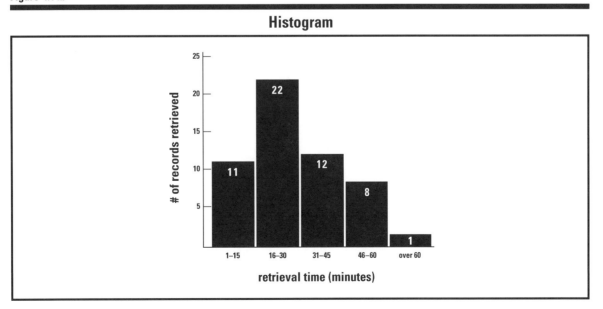

Nominal group technique

Overview

Nominal Group Technique (NGT) is similar to brainstorming, but it goes a step further by incorporating an objective rating system for prioritizing ideas. As in a brainstorming session, CQI team members employing NGT identify as many opportunities for improvement as possible, then they rate all of them to determine which one to pursue first.

When to use NGT

Use NGT when you need to prioritize a list of possible actions, or if you want to identify your department's most significant problem or opportunity.

Putting NGT to work

Step 1

Organize a CQI team.

Step 2

Secure the meeting room and gather materials for recording ideas: a chalkboard or flip chart, writing paper, and pens or pencils.

Step 3

Assemble the group and explain how the NGT works.

Step 4

Introduce the topic to be discussed, and ask a few questions to get the ideas flowing. Consider setting a time limit for this phase of the session, but allot enough time to ensure adequate input.

Step 5

Record all responses on the chalkboard or flip chart.

Step 6

Once the idea-generation phase is complete, cluster similar ideas into categories. For example, if you were discussing reimbursement denials and five responses had something to do with effects coding had on reimbursement, cluster these ideas under the category, "coding."

Step 7

Have participants privately rate each category from one to five, with five being "most important."

Step 8

Tally the individual scores for each category. The category that gets the highest total score is the group's top priority.

Hints:

- Once you've identified your top-priority category, brainstorm ways to address it.
- NGT is a relatively objective way of generating consensus about priorities. It grants equal weight to all opinions, and it reduces the chance that one team member can influence the views of another.

Pareto chart

Overview

The pareto chart is a form of bar graph that displays categories of data in descending order of frequency or significance. It can be used to prioritize options, and is generally used to demonstrate that addressing a single key aspect or defect of a larger system or process will have tremendous impact on that overall system or process.

The pareto chart is named for economist Vilfredo Pareto. He studied the distribution of wealth in 19th-century Italy and found that 80 percent of it was controlled by just 20 percent of the population. That 80–20 breakdown is often referred to as the pareto distribution, and it has given rise to the notion that one can often address 80 percent of the problems in a system by tackling 20 percent of its defects. Quality pioneer Joseph Juran (see Chapter 2, "CQI Basics") developed this CQI tool and named it for Pareto.

When to use a pareto chart

Use a pareto chart when it is crucial that you maximize the effect of limited CQI resources—few people, little time, or a small CQI budget. A pareto chart can help you identify which opportunities for improvement are likely to have the largest impact on your department's performance.

Putting a pareto chart to work

Step 1

Identify an important departmental function and the key activity categories that contribute to it.

Step 2

Establish performance-monitoring mechanisms for each activity category.

Step 3

Track the number of errors—and other indicators of poor performance—that occur within each category.

Step 4

Tally the poor-performance indicators and display the totals—from highest to lowest—in a bar graph (see Figure 4.15).

Figure 4.15

Pareto Chart

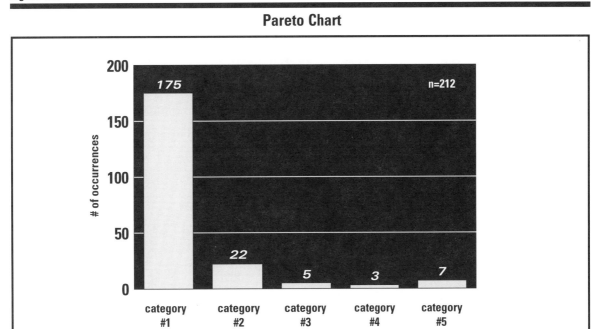

Step 5

If no single category dominates, try recategorizing the raw data you collected until you find a formulation that places a large majority of data in one category.

Step 6

Set the other categories aside and target the dominant one for analysis and improvement.

Hints:

- If you have several problems that are not significant enough to register individually on the chart, clump them together in a group labeled "other."
- The key to using a pareto chart lies in creatively stratifying or categorizing data. To be of use, one category of data needs to be of far greater significance than all others. It doesn't necessarily have to account for 80 percent of the problems or opportunities, but it needs to dominate the others. If your pareto chart doesn't break out this way, recategorize your data until it does.
- Once you've identified a dominant category, the demands of addressing it may still overwhelm your limited CQI resources. If that's the case, narrow the category even further by creating a second-tier pareto chart that isolates sub-categories within that initially dominant category.

The PDCA method

Overview

The PDCA (Plan, Do, Check, Act) method provides an overall framework for CQI—one founded upon a scientific approach to forming and testing hypotheses, monitoring the results of those tests, and, as needed, making data-driven adjustments. The PDCA method was developed in the 1920s by Walter Shewhart, a very early pioneer in statistical quality control. This tool is sometimes called The Deming Cycle, after W. Edwards Deming (see Chapter 2 "CQI Basics"), who popularized its use in Japan.

When to use the PDCA method

The PDCA method provides an effective approach and framework for nearly any CQI initiative; it will govern each phase—from identifying customers and brainstorming problems or opportunities to proposing solutions, implementing them, and monitoring the results (see Figure 4.16). Use it, along with other CQI tools, as a guide for each phase of your program.

Who uses PDCA

Your staff's participation is vital to the PDCA method. They are closest to the processes you'll be addressing, so they are likely to be the best sources for improvement ideas.

Putting PDCA to work

Phase 1: Plan

The planning phase of this tool requires the most effort and time. It involves identifying customers and their needs, identifying areas in which your department is not meeting those needs (or could be meeting them better), and generating improvement proposals. Other CQI tools will be important to the performance-monitoring aspects of this phase. For instance, once you've isolated a process that you'd like to improve, use flow charts, brainstorming, the nominal group technique, pareto charts, surveys, and other tools to evaluate the process and identify opportunities for improvement.

Phase 2: Do

Put your ideas to work during the Do phase of the PDCA method. Once you have settled on improvement proposals, take steps to implement them. You may need to run a small-scale test (a pilot) before launching full-scale initiatives.

Figure 4.16

The PDCA Method

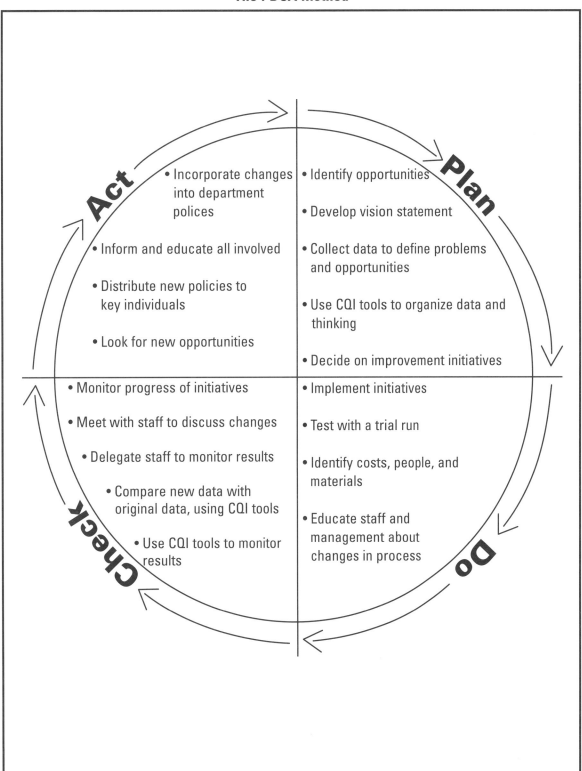

Phase 3: Check

During the Check phase of the PDCA method, you should monitor the results of your improvement initiatives and consider what adjustments may be necessary. Be available to assist staff who are confronting new processes and procedures; they may have questions or offer feedback that can help your evaluation. During the Check phase, meet periodically with staff and the CQI team to discuss how the test is running.

Phase 4: Act

Make adjustments as necessary to the new processes and procedures you've developed. When you are confident they're working effectively, take steps to institutionalize and formalize them by revising departmental policies to incorporate your changes. Train staff and inform other departments about new policies and procedures.

Hints:

- The PDCA method is designed to be a flexible framework for CQI analysis. As new problems or opportunities for improvement arise, launch the process all over again.
- Set quality goals for your department and encourage staff to apply the PDCA method any time they identify opportunities or problems. Regular application of this method is likely to boost your department's efficiency and productivity noticeably.

Pie chart

Overview

Like bar graphs (see page 43), pie charts allow you to compare the relative size of different data sets, or of components parts in the same data set. By doing so, they can help you compare and/or prioritize different aspects of a whole.

When to use a pie chart

Use a pie chart to show how individual aspects or components of some function relate to the whole function. Before and after pie charts are often useful for showing how something has changed as a result of an action taken.

Putting pie charts to work

Step 1

Choose a process that you want to evaluate and determine key indicators for or components of that process.

Step 2

Collect data on the process and organize it into subtotals by indicator or component. A check sheet (see page 54) is a useful tool for organizing such preliminary data. For instance, the sample check sheet below (see Figure 4.17) tracks a facility's monthly delinquent records by doctor.

Figure 4.17

Pie-Chart Data

Chart delinquencies

	Jan.	Feb.	Mar.	Apr.	May	June	6-month total
Dr. Smith	5	10	2	6	8	15	46
Dr. Jones	8	8	7	10	4	2	39
Dr. White	4	4	4	3	6	4	25
Total	17	22	13	19	18	21	110

Step 3

Assign percentages to each indicator subtotal by adding together all the indicator data, dividing each indicator subtotal by the total, and multiplying the result by 100. For instance, on the check sheet below, Dr. Smith accounts for 5 of the 17 chart delinquencies for January. Dividing Dr. Smith's subtotal (5) by the monthly total (17) and multiplying by 100 indicates that he accounted for 29.4 percent of the delinquencies that month.

Step 4

Draw a circle and divide it into proportional segments that are equal to the percentages for each indicator subtotal (see Figure 4.18a).

Step 5

Shade and label each chart wedge and create a legend to identify the each wedge (see Figures 4.18b and 4.18c).

Hint

- If you're creating before-and-after pie charts to illustrate the change in a process due to some action, highlight only the section of the chart relevant to the change.

Figure 4.18a

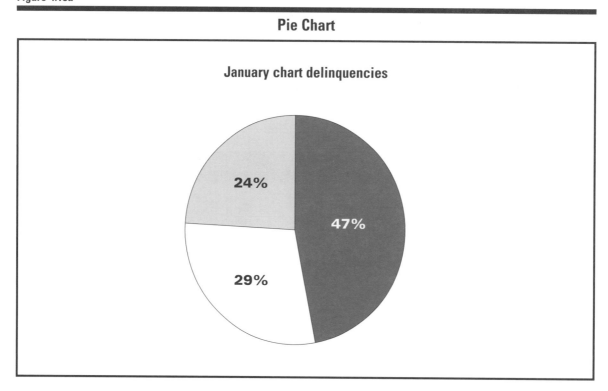

Pie Chart

January chart delinquencies

24%

47%

29%

Figure 4.18b

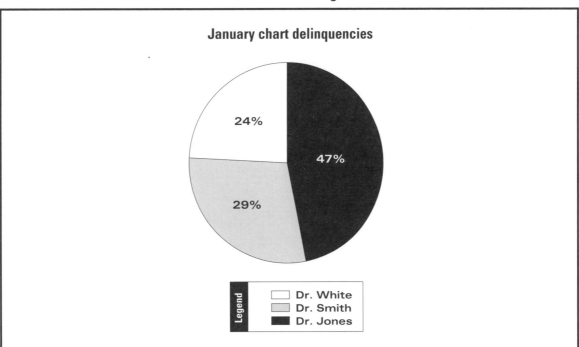

Pie Chart with Legend

January chart delinquencies

24%

47%

29%

Legend
☐ Dr. White
▨ Dr. Smith
■ Dr. Jones

Figure 4.18c

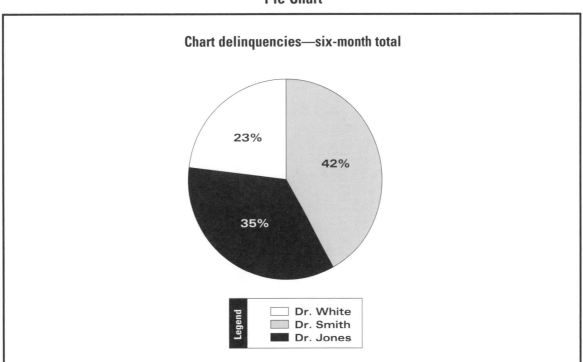

Pie Chart

Chart delinquencies—six-month total

23%

42%

35%

Legend
☐ Dr. White
▨ Dr. Smith
■ Dr. Jones

Radar chart

Overview

A radar chart effectively displays before-and-after data. It measures the strength or weakness of variables and shows how those strengths and weaknesses change over time.

When to use a radar chart

Use a radar chart when you want to demonstrate that progress has been made or that you've lost ground in a specific area. This tool does a good job of showing what lessons your staff has learned and/or what knowledge and skills may be eroding in your department.

Putting a radar chart to work

Step 1

Decide what indicators you'll need to measure. (The radar chart in Figure 4.19 gauges physician confidence in the HIM department, measuring eight indicators.)

Step 2

Draw a circle and divide into equal segments. The number of segments should equal the number of indicators you've chosen.

Step 3

Establish a rating scale for each indicator.

Step 4

Have relevant individuals rate each indicator using the scale you've developed.

Step 5

Average the ratings and post your finding on the segment line for that indicator.

Step 6

Draw a line connecting the posted ratings.

Step 7

Repeat the process at a later date—after implementing improvement initiatives, for instance—and compare the old and new ratings to see where you have improved or where you've regressed. Be sure that the line you use to connect the second set of ratings is different from the one that connects the first set; otherwise you'll have difficulty telling them apart.

Hints

- Points where the second line dips inside the first line indicates regression or a reduction in quality. Points where the second line extends outside the first one indicates improvement.
- Use radar charts to identify opportunities for improvement and/or to help you demonstrate the success of existing improvement initiatives.

Figure 4.19

Radar Chart

Physician assessment of HIM department

Indicators:
A. I have confidence in the HIM department.
B. The HIM staff is cooperative.
C. The HIM department seems committed to improving.
D. The HIM department delivers my charts on time.
E. The HIM department quickly returns charts for signing.
F. The HIM staff understands my needs.
G. I have respect for the HIM department.
H. I enjoy working with HIM employees.

Rating Scale:
1 = disagree strongly
2 = disagree
3 = no opinion
4 = agree
5 = agree strongly

Run chart

Overview

A run chart is a form of line graph that displays the progress of, and variations in, data over time (see Figure 4.20). It allows for quick assessment of performance trends and patterns. For instance, if record delinquencies tend to spike around holidays and vacation periods—when doctors may not be available to sign documents and departments are often short-staffed—a run chart would allow you to spot that trend and plan steps to address it. Run charts track time increments along the horizontal x-axis; frequency is noted along the vertical y-axis.

Figure 4.20

Run Chart

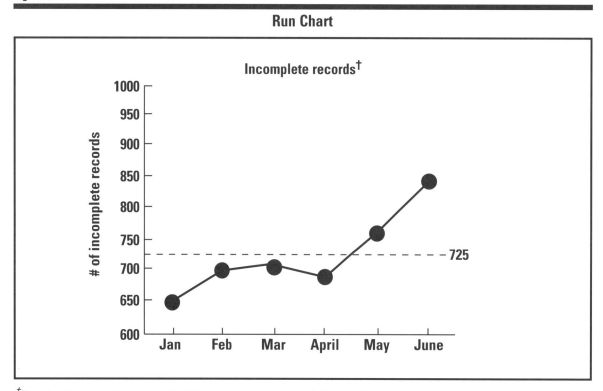

†*The check sheet with raw data for this run chart can be found in Figure 4.5.*

When to use a run chart

Use a run chart when you want to monitor time-related trends and shifts in a process or system. It's a good tool for comparing actual performance to an overall average or to a performance target. It's also a particularly compelling tool for displaying data that reveals the results of an improvement initiative.

Putting run charts to work

Step 1

Select a performance indicator that you'd like to monitor—chart delinquencies, for instance.

Step 2

Settle on a timeframe—chart delinquencies per month, for instance.

Step 3

Establish measurement mechanisms (if you have not already done so) and gather the raw data that you'll be plotting on your run chart. Check sheets (see page 54) are an effective tool for tallying raw data and organizing it into useful categories.

Step 4

Draw your axes, noting months along the horizontal x-axis and frequency indicators along the vertical y-axis (see Figure 4.21a).

Figure 4.21a

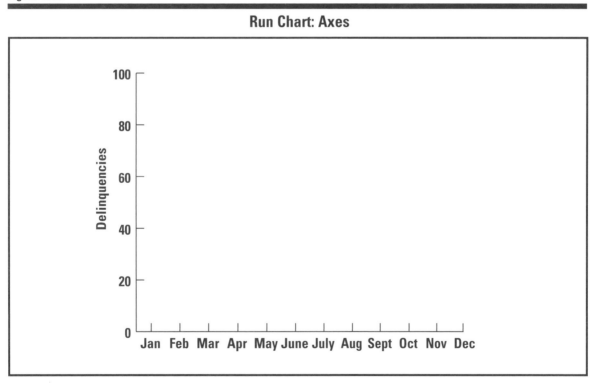

Run Chart: Axes

Step 5

Plot your raw data totals by marking the appropriate x-y intersection points on the run chart. For instance, if you recorded 50 chart delinquencies in January, mark a point directly above "January" on the x-axis and immediately adjacent to "50" on the y-axis (see Figure 4.21b).

Figure 4.21b

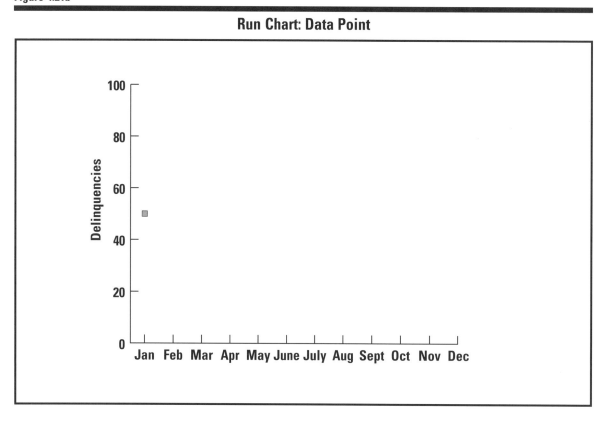

Run Chart: Data Point

Step 6

Once you've plotted all your points, connect them with a line to better highlight the relationships between each point (see Figure 4.21c).

Step 7

To assist your interpretation of the run chart, calculate the average number of chart delinquencies per month. Do this by first adding the totals for each month together and dividing the grand total by the number of months for which data was collected. (For instance, if you noted 400 chart delinquencies over ten months, the average monthly total would be 40 delinquencies.) Find the number along the y-axis that corresponds with the average you have calculated and draw a dotted line out from the axis at that point (see Figure 4.21d).

Figure 4.21c

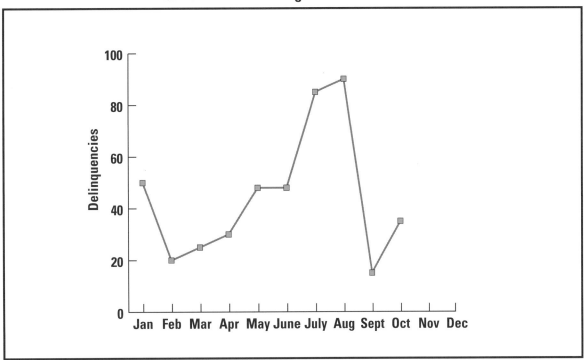

Run Chart: Connecting Plotted Data Points

Figure 4.21d

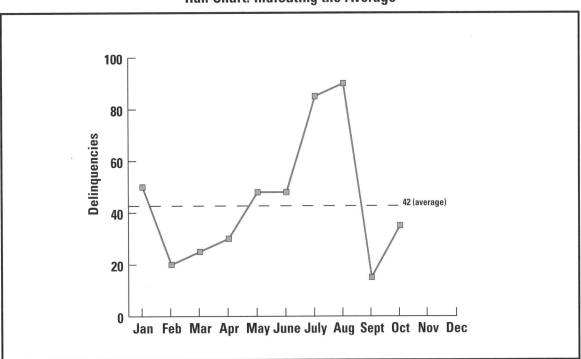

Run Chart: Indicating the Average

Step 8

Look for peaks and valleys on the chart—points at which the monthly totals spike well above, or dip well below, the dotted line marking the average. Your improvement initiative will need to focus on explaining these differentials from the norm.

Hints

- If you want to continue monitoring data after you've drawn the run chart, simply leave enough room along the x-axis to add new time periods and plot new data points.
- If you have departmental performance standards, note the acceptable range on your chart by drawing two dotted lines out from the appropriate point on the y-axis (see Figure 4.21e). This will make it easy to determine the time periods in which staff were operating below or above department standards.
- In addition to displaying data, run charts can provide clues that can help you generate improvement initiatives. For instance, a spike in chart delinquencies during July and August, or during December and January, might be vacation- or holiday-related. Further evaluation would be needed to confirm or disprove this hypothesis.

Figure 4.21e

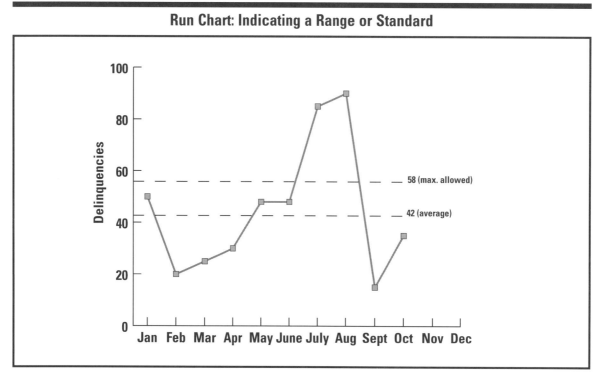

Run Chart: Indicating a Range or Standard

Scatter diagram

Overview

A scatter diagram can help you determine if there is a relationship between two variables—like, for instance, between the age and weight of female patients over 30 (see Figure 4.22). A scatter diagram won't tell you why the variables are related (that would take additional study); it only reveals that a relationship exists.

Figure 4.22

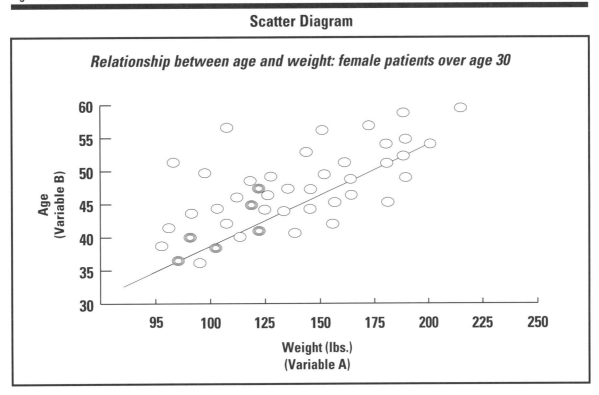

Scatter Diagram

Relationship between age and weight: female patients over age 30

When to use a scatter diagram

Use a scatter diagram any time you need to know whether one aspect of a process or system (one variable) has a predictable effect on another function or process (another variable).

Putting a scatter diagram to work

Step 1

Choose the variables that you want to compare or that you suspect are causally related.

Step 2

Collect data on each. A check sheet is a useful tool for completing this step (see Figure 4.23, below, and refer to page 54).

Figure 4.23

Plotting a Scatter Diagram from Check-Sheet Data

Patient Name	Age	Weight
1. M. Smith	48	150
2. J. Jones	40	125
3. B. Davis	38	100
4. F. Bailey	35	145
5. J. Nu	58	200
6. A. Wood	41	105
7. M. Foley	50	180
Etc.	. . .	. . .
50. M. Madden	42	142

Step 3

Note the highest and lowest values for each variable.

Step 4

Draw axes for each variable. Note the data-scale for each (your scales should begin with the lowest values noted during step 3 and extend at least to the highest values).

Step 5

Plot each data point by indicating where their two measurements intersect on the diagram. For instance, to plot data for the first patient on the check sheet in Figure 4.23, you'd mark the point above "150" on the x-axis and adjacent to "48" on the y-axis. If you plot the same data point more than once, circle that mark.

Step 6

Once you plot your data points, evaluate the pattern of marks on the diagram to determine whether a correlation between the variables exists. For instance:

- The diagram indicates a positive correlation if the data points are clustered together in a relatively tight band that extends from the lower left toward the upper right (see Figure 4.24a). A positive correlation means that an increase in the x-axis variable prompts an increase in the y-axis variable.

- A negative correlation between the variables exists if the data points are clustered together in a band that extends from upper left to lower right (see Figure 4.24b). A negative correlation indicates that an increase in the x-axis variable will produce a decrease in the y-axis variable.
- If the data points are scattered randomly across the diagram, no correlation exists between the variables (see Figure 4.24c)—that is, a change in one does not produce a predictable effect on the other.

Figure 4.24a

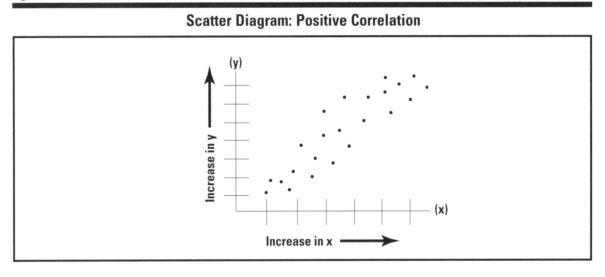

Scatter Diagram: Positive Correlation

Figure 4.24b

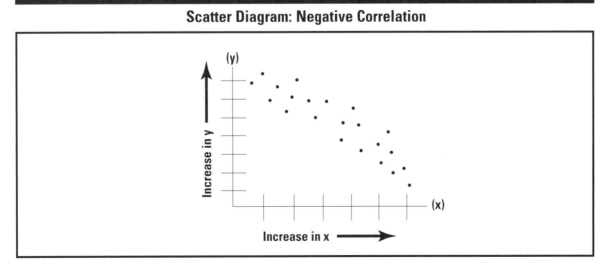

Scatter Diagram: Negative Correlation

Figure 4.24c

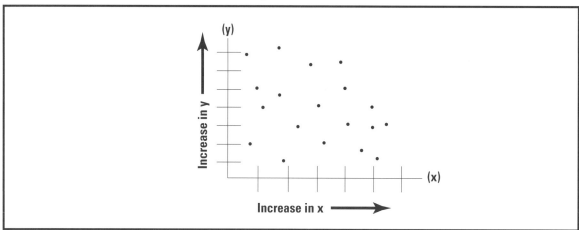

Scatter Diagram: No Correlation

- Now and then, you'll come across a cluster pattern like the one shown in Figure 4.24d. This pattern indicates that the correlation between your variables shifts; the y-axis variable increases along with the x-axis variable until you reach a particular point (the point of diminishing returns, so to speak), at which time the correlation becomes negative. Generally this means that a process has reached a key threshold; one that, if you were considering improvement initiatives, you'd need to understand.

Figure 4.24d

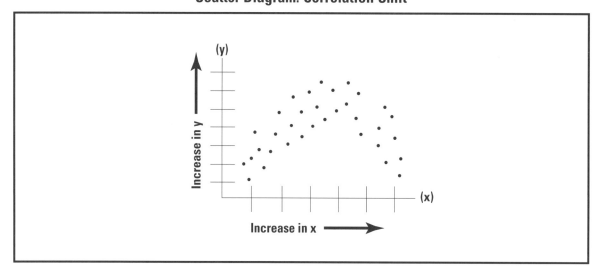

Scatter Diagram: Correlation Shift

Continuous Quality Improvement for Health Information Management

Hints

- Do not connect the plotted points on a scatter diagram—look only at the cluster pattern that they create.
- Scatter diagrams are most effective if you have a lot of data points. Otherwise, it's difficult to discern a clear cluster pattern.
- Sometimes a scatter diagram conveys a correlation that, in reality, does not exist because the variables that you are measuring are actually under the influence of a third variable. For instance, a town may see a rise in milk consumption alongside an increase in the number of children playing little league baseball. A scatter diagram that displays those variables might suggest a relationship when, in fact, both increases are actually due to an increase in the population of children living in the town. To avoid misleading results, choose your variables carefully; logic should tell you that they're causally related.
- To use scatter-diagram data effectively, it's important to move beyond simply identifying a correlation between two variables. You need to figure out why the relationship exists.

Survey/questionnaire

Overview

A written survey or questionnaire allows CQI teams to gather specific feedback on a process or issue from a large group of people. Surveys and questionnaires are often more objective than interviews because the wording of questions can't be changed, and other outside influences are eliminated (e.g., an interviewer's tone or body language). Also, since every respondent is asked to answer an identical set of questions, this tool elicits feedback that can be analyzed statistically.

When to use a survey/questionnaire

Use a written survey/questionnaire (see Figure 4.25) when your CQI team needs feedback from more people than can be easily interviewed, or when you need to present questions objectively and/or in a consistent fashion to all respondents. Surveys are also useful when your team is planning to ask the same group a series of questions several times (perhaps to gauge shifts in attitude as a process unfolds or evolves) and needs to ensure that the wording and delivery of the questions are consistent each time.

Putting a survey/questionnaire to work

Step 1

The first step in developing a survey is to identify what you need to know. Think about the product, service, or function that your team is analyzing, then develop questions designed to elicit the information you need.

Step 2

Identify your internal and external customers and decide how many you'll need to survey to get an adequate cross-section of viewpoints.

Step 3

Draft your questions carefully to ensure objectivity. Try to avoid using language that leads respondents to answer a particular way or that reveals the biases of the questioner.

Step 4

Ask people from your department to test the survey. If they find the questions or directions hard to follow, or if their responses don't generate useful information, redesign the survey.

Figure 4.25

HIM Survey of Physicians

Please take a moment to complete the following survey. Use the rating system indicated. If you have additional comments, please note them at the end of the survey. Thank you.

Rating system
1 = poor   2 = adequate   3 = good   4 = excellent

Rating	
_____	1. Rate the adequacy of the equipment that the HIM department provides (dictation machines, etc.)
_____	2. Rate the HIM department's turnaround time for:
_____	• transcription
	• record retrieval
_____	3. Rate the HIM department's accuracy for:
_____	• transcription
	• record retrieval
_____	4. Rate the utility of the dictation system
_____	5. Rate the HIM staff in terms of:
_____	• friendliness
_____	• cooperation
_____	• hours of service
	• efficiency

Comments: _____

_____

May we contact you? ❑ Yes   ❑ No

Signature: _____

Name: _____ Extension or pager number: _____

Step 5

Once you're satisfied with the survey format, distribute enough questionnaires to ensure an adequate response rate. If you want at least 50 responses, for instance, you might consider distributing 100 surveys. Include a letter telling potential respondents the reason for the survey and explaining why you would like their input (see Figure 4.26). If there's a response deadline, alert them to it.

Step 6

Analyze the surveys when you get them back. You might use a check sheet to tally responses. Other tools—cause-and-effect diagrams, pareto charts, and scatter diagrams, for instance—can also assist your analysis.

Hints

- Keep surveys simple and to the point. Asking too many questions, or asking complex questions, may hurt your response rate.
- Give everyone an identical survey or your data will be corrupt.
- To ensure the consistency of the information you gather, consider having respondents choose from a predetermined set of answers (this is known as the range/rating method). For example, a questionnaire surveying doctors about records retrieval might include the following:
  > How often are your records requests filled within an hour?
  > 1 = always
  > 2 = most of the time
  > 3 = about half the time
  > 4 = now and then
  > 5 = never
- If you need a high response rate, send a cover letter to your respondent pool encouraging participation. You may even want to offer incentives (e.g., a small reward or gift) to respondents who return completed surveys on time (see Figure 4.26).
- Make sure you give people enough time to fit the survey into their schedules.
- Do not over-survey one group of respondents. They may get annoyed.

Figure 4.26

Sample Cover Letter for HIM Survey of Physicians

Dear Dr. _____:

As part of the HIM Department's ongoing commitment to quality improvement, we are sur-veying key internal customers and would appreciate your candid feedback concerning HIM services. Please take a few minutes to answer each question on the enclosed survey so we may organize our services to better assist your patient-care activities.

Please indicate in the appropriate space if we may contact you for clarification of your answers. All completed surveys (with signatures) will be entered in a drawing for a dictation machine.

Thank you for your assistance.

Sincerely,

HIM Director

Chapter 5:
Case Studies

Chapter 5: Case Studies

Introduction

This chapter contains four in-depth examples of how organizations have used CQI principles and techniques to improve key HIM-related functions and processes. In each one, data was the basis for action, and we give specific examples of how data was gathered, organized, analyzed, and displayed. We have included the case studies for three reasons: 1) They provide practical examples of CQI in action; 2) They may guide improvement initiatives at your facility; and 3) They demonstrate how some organizations have addressed the issue of employee resistance to change.

To better link the case studies to other chapters throughout the book, we include a list at the end of each one that highlights the CQI tools that were discussed and applied. Where appropriate, we also include cross references that point you toward supporting or complementary sections of this book. We hope these cases are both helpful and useful as you seek to establish a CQI culture within your department or organization.

Vital Statistics

Organization: Fairview Health Services

Type: Integrated Delivery System

Location: Minneapolis, MN

Facilities: 21 ambulatory clinics (Fairview Clinics); 4 acute-care campuses

Caseload: 40,000 patients per month (clinics only)

Ambulatory Clinics Standardize Documentation and Posting

In an age of mega-mergers and far-flung healthcare networks, many organizations face the difficult task of integrating systems and standardizing procedures across different locations and care settings. Here's how one network of ambulatory clinics used CQI to confront that challenge.

Overview

In 1996, Minneapolis-based Fairview Clinics convened a CQI team to examine its procedures for documenting and posting the services that patients receive in its 21 ambulatory-care clinics. As the clinic network, which is affiliated with Fairview Health Services, grew over the years, the forms and procedures associated with documentation and posting remained largely distinct at each site. But for the doctors, nurses, and other staff who float between locations, the lack of standardization was confusing. As a result, the quality of the information that they recorded for billing purposes suffered. Health information manager LaVonne Wieland and regional administrator Judy Treharne initiated the CQI process, believing that standardizing the documentation and posting process across clinic locations would reduce confusion and costly rework. They also felt that, by improving the accuracy and efficiency of documentation and posting, standardization would increase reimbursement.

Getting started

After securing the support of key senior management, Treharne and Wieland recruited a core team to plan a CQI initiative. They began meeting in February 1996, with the intention of having a standardized process up and running by April 1997.

The core team launched the planning phase of the initiative with a brainstorming session to identify the products and services associated with documentation and posting (see Figure 1a) and the "customers" who used those products (see Figure 1b). This brainstorming, said Wieland, clarified what was at stake and provided the raw materials for a vision statement. That statement outlined their broad objectives and was designed, like a fixed point on the horizon, to keep the yearlong initiative pointed in the right direction.

Figure 1a

HIM Products and Services

❏ Date—transaction level and summary level
❏ A bill or statement—i.e., HCFA 1500
❏ Posted batches
❏ Data associated with outcome management
❏ Charge tickets

Figure 1b

HIM Customers

❏ Patients   ❏ Physicians
❏ Payers   ❏ Nurses and medical assistants
❏ Central business office   ❏ Laboratory technicians
❏ Data-entry staff   ❏ Radiology technicians
❏ Coders   ❏ Receptionists

The charge ticket

A form known as the "charge ticket" lay at the heart of Fairview's standardization efforts. At the beginning of each patient encounter, office staff print a charge ticket and label it with demographic and insurance information. During the encounter, doctors, nurses, lab technicians, and other personnel use the form to log the services rendered. Once an encounter is complete, coders compare the services noted on the charge ticket with the information in the medical record. If the documentation in the record supports the charge ticket, a bill for the encounter is issued.

When Fairview Clinics launched its CQI initiative, all 21 locations used a different charge ticket. The lack of consistency, said Wieland, often led staff to complete charge tickets incorrectly, or created situations in which charge-ticket notations were not adequately documented in the patient record. At best, she explained, mistakes and poor documentation delayed the billing process. But even more concerning was the likely possibility that staff had been failing to record some services altogether, which would mean Fairview was under-billing for some encounters. Any successful effort to improve documentation and posting, therefore, had to involve development of a standard charge-ticket format.

Divide and conquer

Having isolated charge-ticket format as a key focus of its CQI initiative, the core team began to consider charge-ticket processing. Meeting roughly every two weeks, the team had, by late March, isolated three key stages of processing that seemed likely to benefit from examination: 1) registration/labeling; 2) entry of services; and 3) data entry and posting.

To expedite data collection and analysis, the core team established four subgroups—one to standardize charge-ticket format, which Wieland led, and three others to examine each key stage of charge-ticket processing. To guide the work of each subgroup, the core team created a grid (see Figure 2) that identified key "inputs" (materials and information to be analyzed) and "suppliers" (sources where those materials and information were available).

Subgroup on charge-ticket format

Wieland says her subgroup's mission was really two-pronged: 1) create a charge ticket that staff would recognize and understand—no matter what location they were working in; and 2) design the ticket to minimize the potential for mistakes and miscommunication of information. The first goal was relatively unambiguous; the team addressed it by evaluating charge tickets from each location to identify and eliminate points of difference.

Figure 2

CQI Inputs and Suppliers

CORE PROCESS	Create a Charge Ticket	Labels on Charge Tickets	Services Documented on Charge Ticket	Coding
INPUTS	• Old charge ticket • Reports from query (system) • Coding books	• Account maintenance • Scheduling • Labels, printers PACE	• Service provided • Charge ticket • Supplies (medical)	• Books, manuals • Diagnosis • Charge ticket • Documentation of service • Transcription
SUPPLIERS	• Clinic • Regulatory requirements	• Patient • Payer • Physician • Companies • Pt. information supervisors • Practice management subcommittee • Information services • Schedulers/ receptionists • Business-office staff • Referral department	• Provider • Lab and x-ray • Business office and nursing • Regulatory requirements • Hospitals, nursing homes, and reference lab • Other clinics	• Regulatory requirements • Provider • Nursing • Lab/x-ray • Business office
TEAM MEMBERS	L. Wieland (lead) J. P. Minge S. Kroening D. Scholl C. Garner	K. Gray (lead) C. Screeden D. Vrieze K. Gunderson B. McMenomy V. Newton	C. Screeden (co-lead) L. Wieland (co-lead) C. Garner S. Kroening B. McMenomy J. P. Minge M. Koenke Representative from lab, x-ray, nursing	C. Screeden (co-lead) L. Wieland (co-lead) C. Garner S. Kroening J. P. Minge Representatives from lab, x-ray, nursing Input from coder network group

Since the forms are used for the same purpose in each clinic—to capture and code information related to patient demographics and the services performed during a single encounter—the team quickly determined that its challenge lay in standardizing the layout. They settled on a format that reserved the top quarter of the page for ICD-9 codes and a label containing basic information on the patient and the encounter. The rest of the page was divided into three columns. Initially, the left-hand side was reserved for more details on the patient and his or her visit, the center column tracked clinic services, and the right-hand column was for lab services (see Figure 3a). Wieland says the team eventually decided to create a separate charge ticket for lab services, because the rules and regulations that govern coding for those services made it too complicated to include everything on one form. After deleting lab services, the team expanded the section set aside for clinic services (see Figure 3b, page 107).

The second goal of the subgroup on charge-ticket format, designing a form that would minimize mistakes and miscommunication of information, was not so straightforward. Here, the team got help from the subgroup examining the procedures for entering services on the charge ticket. That team had developed a survey, which revealed, among other things, that staff were unhappy with the amount of information that had to be handwritten on charge tickets. Wieland's format subgroup realized that dependence on handwritten completion made errors more likely, and may even have been discouraging staff from noting all services performed during encounters. So subgroup members decided to reduce dependence on handwritten information by printing the most common clinic services and codes directly on the standard form.

Ironically, printing codes and services on the charge ticket made it impossible to create a single form for use in all clinics; each location's menu of common services varied just enough to make a comprehensive list unwieldy. However, the general categories of services were, with minor exception, identical. So, the team compromised, creating a form with category headings that were, in large part, standard (i.e., procedures, diagnostic tests, supplies, injections, immunizations, etc.), but that allowed individual clinics to choose specific services to list as subheadings (see Figures 4a & 4b, pages 108–109). The result was a standard format that would be familiar to all employees, but that also had the flexibility to be as useful as possible for each clinic.

Figure 3a

Draft Charge-Ticket Format

Patient Name_____

Birth Date____ /____ /____ Account Type_____

Doctor #_____ Location_____

Visit Date____ /____ /____

Account #_____

Case ID_____ (work comp only)

Coder Use Only:

ICD9   1._____   3._____

        2._____   4._____

1 MD only

2 nurse only

3 lab, x-ray only, supplies

auto / liab. injury date_____ /_____ /_____

Diagnosis: 1._____   2._____   3._____   4._____

MD	CODE	DX	OFFICE VISITS
			NEW PATIENT
	99201		problem focused
	99202		exp. problem focused
	99203		detailed
	99204		comprehensive/ mod. complexity
	99205		comprehensive/ high complexity
			ESTABLISHED PATIENT
	99211		nurse only – minimal
	99212		problem focused
	99213		exp. problem focused
	99214		detailed
	99215		comprehensive/ high complexity

MD	CODE	DX	PREVENTIVE MEDICINE
			NEW PATIENT
	99381		under 1 year
	99382		1–4 years
	99383		5–11 years
	99384		12–17 years
	99385		18–39 years
	99386		40–64 years
	99387		65 years and over
			ESTABLISHED PATIENT
	99391		under 1 year
	99392		1–4 years
	99393		5–11 years
	99394		12–17 years
	99395		18–39 years
	99396		40–64 years
	99397		65 years and over

MD	CODE	DX	CONSULTATIONS
			OUTPATIENT/OFFICE
REFERRING MD:			
			CONFIRMATORY

MD	CODE	DX	PROCEDURES

MD	CODE	DX	SUPPLIES

MD	CODE	DX	INJECTIONS

MD	CODE	DX	IMMUNIZATIONS

MD	CODE	DX	X-RAY

MD	CODE	DX	INHOUSE LAB

MD	CODE	DX	REFERENCE LAB

MD	CODE	DX	MISCELLANEOUS

Figure 3b

Draft Format (no lab information)

Patient Name_____

Birth Date____ /____ /____ Account Type_____

Doctor #_____ Location_____

Visit Date____ /____ /____

Account #_____

Case ID_____ (work comp only)

_____

Coder Use Only:

ICD9 1._____ 3._____
       2._____ 4._____

1 MD only
2 nurse only
3 lab, x-ray only, supplies

auto / liab. injury date_____ /_____ /_____

Diagnosis: 1._____ 2._____ 3._____ 4._____

MD	CODE	DX	OFFICE VISITS
			NEW PATIENT
	99201		problem focused
	99202		exp. problem focused
	99203		detailed
	99204		comprehensive/ mod. complexity
	99205		comprehensive/ high complexity
			ESTABLISHED PATIENT
	99211		nurse only – minimal
	99212		problem focused
	99213		exp. problem focused
	99214		detailed
	99215		comprehensive/ high complexity

MD	CODE	DX	PREVENTIVE MEDICINE
			NEW PATIENT
	99381		under 1 year
	99382		1–4 years
	99383		5–11 years
	99384		12–17 years
	99385		18–39 years
	99386		40–64 years
	99387		65 years and over
			ESTABLISHED PATIENT
	99391		under 1 year
	99392		1–4 years
	99393		5–11 years
	99394		12–17 years
	99395		18–39 years
	99396		40–64 years
	99397		65 years and over

MD	CODE	DX	GLOBAL SERVICES

MD	CODE	DX	CONSULTATIONS
			OUTPATIENT/OFFICE
			REFERRING MD:
			CONFIRMATORY

MD	CODE	DX	PROCEDURES

MD	CODE	DX	DIAGNOSTIC TESTS

MD	CODE	DX	CARDIAC EVENT MONITOR

MD	CODE	DX	CYTOLOGY/PATHOLOGY

MD	CODE	DX	SUPPLIES

MD	CODE	DX	INJECTIONS

MD	CODE	DX	IMMUNIZATIONS

MD	CODE	DX	X-RAY

Figure 4a

Standard Format with Customized Subheadings

Patient Name_____

Birth Date____ /____ /____ Account Type_____

Doctor #_____ Location_____

Visit Date____ /____ /____ Account #_____

Case ID_____ (work comp only)

Coder Use Only:

ICD9   1. _____   3. _____

         2. _____   4. _____

1. MD only / 2. nurse only / 3. lab, x-ray only, supplies

Diagnosis: 1._____ 2._____ 3._____ 4._____ auto / liab. injury date____ /____ /____

MD	CODE	MOD	DX	OFFICE VISITS
				NEW PATIENT
	99201			problem focused
	99202			exp. problem focused
	99203			detailed
	99204			comprehensive-mod. complexity
	99205			comprehensive-high complexity
	99025			new pt. with procedure
				ESTABLISHED PATIENT
	99211			nurse only – minimal
	99212			problem focused
	99213			exp. problem focused
	99214			detailed
	99215			comprehensive-high complexity
	99450			DOT physical (incl. UA)
	4008			FAA physical
	8810			pre-placement exam

MD	CODE	DX	PREVENTIVE MEDICINE	MD	CODE	DX
			NEW PATIENT		ESTABLISHED	
	99381		under 1 year		99391	
	99382		1–4 years		99392	
	99383		5–11 years		99393	
	99384		12–17 years		99394	
	99385		18–39 years		99395	
	99386		40–64 years		99396	
	99387		65 years and over		99397	

MD	CODE	DX	GLOBAL SERVICES
	4005		fracture care
	99024		post-op visit

MD	CODE	MOD	DX	CONSULTATIONS
				OUTPATIENT/OFFICE
REFERRING MD:				
	99241			problem focused
	99242			exp. problem focused
	99243			detailed
	99244			comprehensive - mod. complexity
	99245			comprehensive - high complexity

MD	CODE	DX	DIAGNOSTIC TESTS
	93000		EKG
	93010		EKG, interp. & report
	93224		holter monitor
	94010		spirometry
	94060		pre & post treatment
	93015		stress test
	94150		vital capacity, measure only

MD	CODE	MOD	DX	PROCEDURES
	46600			anoscopy
	92551			audiometry
	17340			cryotherapy for acne
	17110			destruction molluscum; flat warts
				retreatment (use E/M)
	4300			destruction skin lesion
				(plantar wart)
	4301x			2-14: specify #
	4302			15 or more
	69210			ear irrigation
	58100			endometrial biopsy
				I & D abscess
	10060			simple, single
	10061			complicated, multiple
	20610			injection joint major
				drug
	11200			removal skin tag 15 or less
	11201x			ea. addit'l 10: specify #
	45330			sigmoidoscopy, diagnostic
	45331			with biopsy

MD	CODE	DX	CARDIAC EVENT MONITOR
	4200		complete pkg.
	8648		hook-up only
	8609		monitoring only
	4201		phys. read only

MD	CODE	DX	CYTOLOGY/PATHOLOGY
	2864		pap smear
	1916		pap handling
	1914		surgical tissue
	2888		level 1
	2890		level 2
	2892		level 3
	2894		level 4
	2896		level 5

MD	CODE	DX	SUPPLIES
			splint: specify

MD	CODE	DX	INJECTIONS
	90782		admin. subq./intramusc.
	95115		allergy - single
	95117		allergy - multiple
	8093		demerol per 100 mg
	8550		depo provera 150 mg (contraceptive)
	8267		depo testosterone 200 mg
	8199		gold up to 50 mg

MD	CODE	DX	INJECTIONS (cont.)
	8145		imforon 2 cc
	1650		mantoux (PPD)
	8040		penicillin 1.2 mil
	8165		phenergan up to 50 mg
	8215		vitamin B-12 up to 1000 mg

MD	CODE	DX	IMMUNIZATIONS
	90718		chicken pox
	90725		cholera
	90702		DT
	90700		DTaP
	90720		DTP/HIB
	90724		flu vaccine
	8650		admin. (if no E/M) (Medicare only)
	90730		hepatitis A
	90744		hep. B < 11 years
	90745		11-19 years
	90746		> 20 years
	8660		admin. (if no E/M) (Medicare only)
	90737		HIB
	90733		meningococcal
	90707		MMR
	90732		pneumococcal
	8655		admin. (if no E/M) (Medicare only)
	90712		polio - oral
	90713		polio - injectable
	90703		tetanus
			typhoid

MD	CODE	DX	X-RAY
	74020		abdomen - flat & upright
	74000		abdomen - KUB
	73610		ankle, 3 views minimum
	72052		cervical spine, complete
	71010		chest
	71020		chest PA & lateral
	71101		chest and ribs
	73070		elbow - AP and lateral
	73550		femur
	73140		finger, 3 views
	73630		foot, 3 views minimum
	73090		forearm – AP and lateral
	73130		hand – 3 views minimum
	73650		heel – 2 views minimum
	73510		hip – 2 views minimum
	73060		humerus – 2 views minimum
	73560		knee – AP and lateral
	73562		knee – AP and lateral w/ oblique(s)

Figure 4b

Standard Format with Customized Subheadings

Patient Name_____

Birth Date____ /____ /____ Account Type_____

Doctor #_____ Location_____

Visit Date____ /____ /____ Account #_____

Case ID_____ (work comp only)

Coder Use Only:
ICD9   1._____   3._____
2._____   4._____
1. MD only / 2. nurse only / 3. lab, x-ray only, supplies

Diagnosis: 1._____ 2._____ 3._____ 4._____   auto / liab. injury date____ /____ /____

MD	CODE	MOD	DX	OFFICE VISITS
				NEW PATIENT
	99201			problem focused
	99202			exp. problem focused
	99203			detailed
	99204			comprehensive-mod. complexity
	99205			comprehensive-high complexity
	99025			new patient with procedure
				ESTABLISHED PATIENT
	99211			minimal
	99212			problem focused
	99213			exp. problem focused
	99214			detailed
	99215			comprehensive-high complexity
	99450			DOT physical (incl. UA)
	8810			pre-placement exam

MD	CODE	DX	PREVENTIVE MEDICINE	MD	CODE	DX
			NEW PATIENT			ESTABLISHED
	99381		under 1 year		99391	
	99382		1–4 years		99392	
	99383		5–11 years		99393	
	99384		12–17 years		99394	
	99385		18–39 years		99395	
	99386		40–64 years		99396	
	99387		65 years and over		99397	

MD	CODE	DX	GLOBAL SERVICES
	99024		post-op visit
	4000		prenatal visit
	4004		postpartum visit

MD	CODE	MOD	DX	RISK FACTOR COUNSELING
	99401			15 minutes
	99402			30 minutes

MD	CODE	MOD	DX	CONSULT OFFICE/OUTPATIENT
REQUESTING MD:				
	99241			problem focused
	99242			exp. problem focused
	99243			detailed

MD	CODE	MOD	DX	DIAGNOSTIC TESTS
	92552			audiometry
	93000			EKG
	93224			holter monitor
	94760			pulse oximetry
	93015			stress test
	94010			spirometry
	94060			pre and post bronchodilation
	92567			tympanometry

MD	CODE	MOD	DX	PROCEDURES
				application of:
				( ) cast ( ) splint
	10160			aspirate abscess, cyst, hematoma
	11100			biopsy skin, subq tissue,
				single lesion
	57452			colposcopy
	11720			debridement of nails: 1-5
	17110			destruction molluscum; flat warts:
				to 15 (retreatment, charge as E/M)
	4300			destruction skin lesion
				(plantar wart)
	4301			each addl. up to 14: specify #
	69210			ear irrigation (one or both ears)
	17200			electrosurg. destr. of skin tags:
				1-15
	58100			endometrial biopsy
				excise skin lesion
				( ) benign ( ) malig.
				site: size: cm
				site: size: cm
	45330			flex sigmoidoscopy
	10060			I & D skin abscess: simple, single
	10061			I & D skin abscess: compl. or mult.
				inject/aspirate joint, bur. gang cyst
	20600			small (fingers, toes)
	20605			medium (wrist, elbow, ankle)
	20610			large (shoulder, hip, knee)
	20550			tendon sheath, ligament trig. point
				drug: dose:
	53670			insert urinary catheter, simple
	8808			nail trimming, routine root care
	94640			nebulizer tx., acute airway obstr.
	11050			pare corn, callus, wart: sing. lesion
	10120			remove nail plate: simple, single
	11200			remove skin tags: 15 or less
				repair lacer. ( ) simple ( ) layer
				site: size:
				shave removal, benign skin lesion
				site: size: cm
				site: size: cm
	55250			vasectomy
	8540			surgery tray, vasectomy

MD	CODE	MOD	DX	SUPPLIES
				cast supplies: (specify)
	8280			elastic bandage (ace)
	8005			surgery tray, small
				other supplies

MD	CODE	MOD	DX	CYTOPATHOLOGY
	2864			pap smear
	1916			pap handling
	8635			pap handling - Medicare/MA
	1914			surgical tissue handling
	2892			level 3 pathology
	2894			level 4 pathology

MD	CODE	MOD	DX	INJECTIONS/AGENTS
	90782			admin. subq./IM inject.
	90788			admin. IM antibiotic
	95115			allergy inject. - single
	95117			allergy inject. - multiple
	8575			aristospan mg
	8215			B-12 to 1000 mcg
	8040			bicillin CR 1.2 MU
	8055			bicillin LA 1.2 MU
	8910			celestone mg
	8093			demerol mg
				depo medrol mg
	8550			depo provera 150 mg (contracep.)
				depo testosterone
	8170			kenalog mg
	8565			rocephin mg
	1650			TB, intradermal-PPD

MD	CODE	MOD	DX	IMMUNIZATIONS
	90716			chicken pox
	90702			DT (peds)
	90700			DTaP
	90721			DTaP/HIB
	90701			DTP
	90720			DTP/HIB
	90730			hepatitis A
	90744			hepatitis B, age 0-10
	90745			11-19 years
	90746			20 years and over
	8660			Medicare admin. no E/M visit
	90707			MMR
	90732			pneumococcal
	8655			Medicare admin. no E/M visit
	90712			polio - oral
	90713			polio - injectable
	90718			td (adult)
	90703			tetanus toxoid

MD	CODE	MOD	DX	X-RAY
	74000			abdomen - KUB
	74020			abdomen - flat & upright
	73610			ankle, 3 views minimum
	73600			ankle, AP and lateral

Subgroups on charge-ticket processing

As the subgroup on charge-ticket format was producing a form for use in each clinic, the other three subgroups focused on standardizing the ways each facility handled the charge ticket. Using detailed flow charts, for instance, the registration subgroup was able to streamline the process used, in all but one clinic, to generate patient labels for the charge ticket (see Figures 5a & 5b). The exception, Oxboro Clinic, is Fairview's largest and treats roughly 11,000 of the 40,000 patients who visit the clinic network each month. To manage that caseload, Oxboro was forced to create an account maintenance department (see Figures 5c & 5d, pages 113–115), which unavoidably added extra steps to its registration process. Other than these slight variations at Oxboro, however, the team created a standardized model for registration that each clinic is adopting.

Likewise, flow charts were a valuable tool for the team examining how services are entered on a charge ticket and documented in a patient's chart. Each time the team's flow charts identified points where the process seemed to stall, members surveyed people involved in that stage of the process. By asking those individuals and departments what they did with the charge ticket or chart and, more significantly, whether they really needed to see those documents, the subgroup discovered a number of unnecessary steps in the process. After addressing those situations and combining their flow-chart and survey analysis with that of the data entry and posting group, the team was able to develop more streamlined procedures for completing and posting the new charge ticket (see Figure 6, page 116).

Maintaining the momentum

As planned, the Fairview Clinics CQI team introduced the new charge ticket and the improved procedures for completing it in the spring of 1997. Wieland said it wasn't uncommon for clinics to resist some of the changes—at least initially. But she said that resistance was surprisingly short-lived, and feedback is now largely positive.

Individual clinics have suggested alterations and changes to the new charge ticket, which Wieland is responsible for considering. She says she assesses all requests for change and does her best to be accommodating. But she also guards the now-standardized procedures carefully and won't approve alterations that can't be absorbed across clinic sites.

Figure 5a

Existing- and New-Patient Registration Process

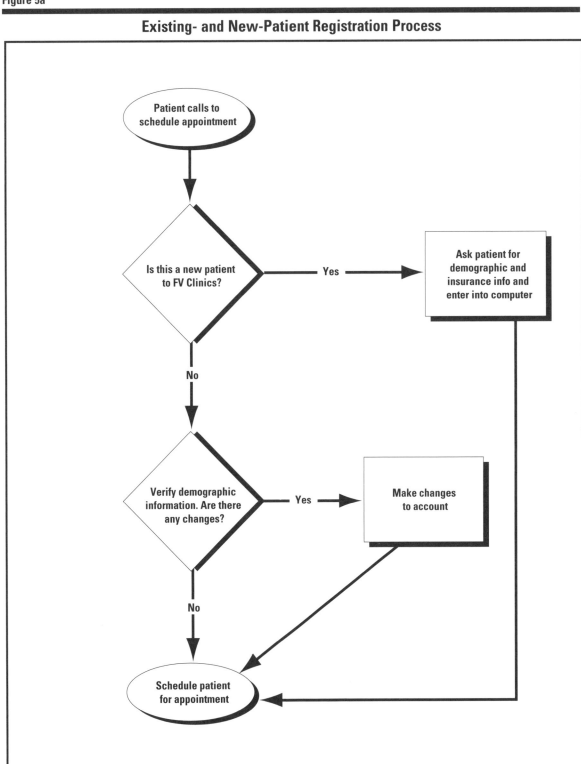

Figure 5b

Patient Check-In Process

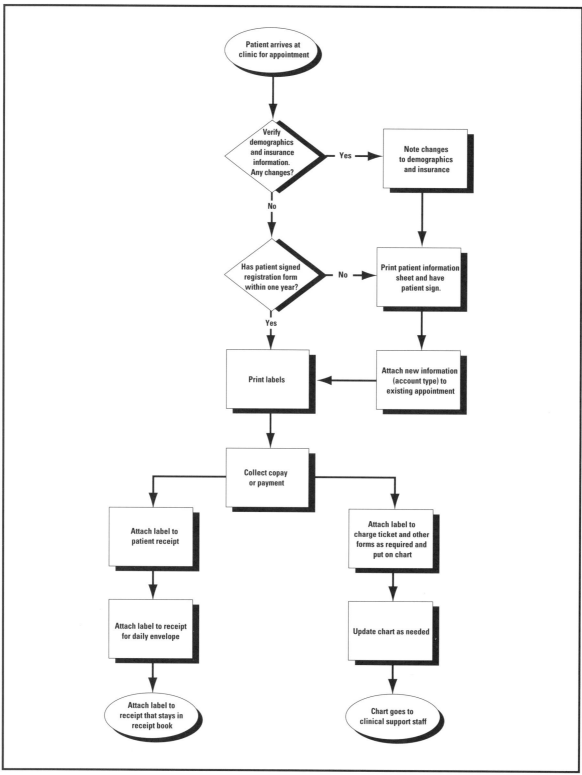

Figure 5c

Oxboro Clinic: Existing- and New-Patient Registration Process

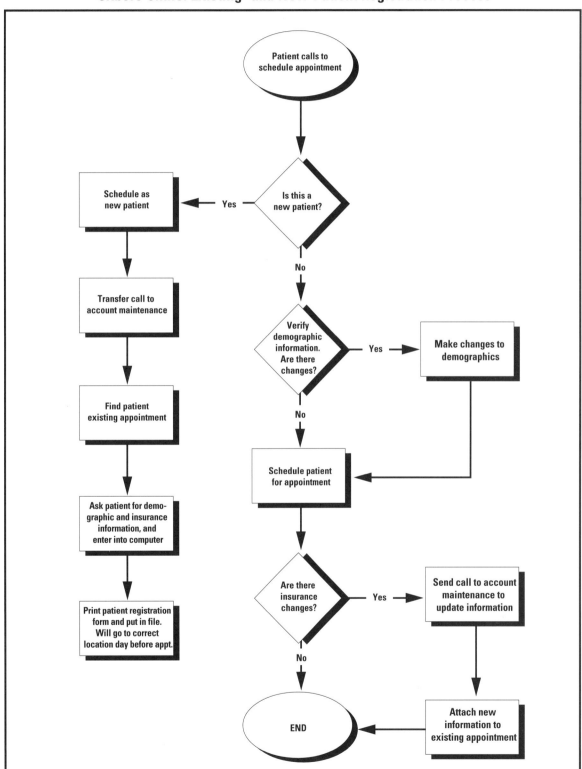

Figure 5d

Oxboro Clinic: Patient Check-In Process

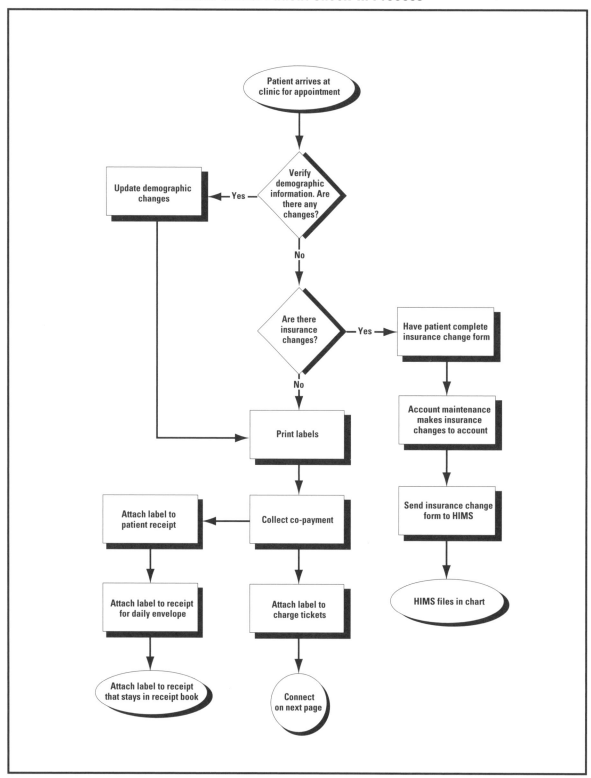

Figure 5d (cont.)

Oxboro Clinic: Patient Check-In Process (cont.)

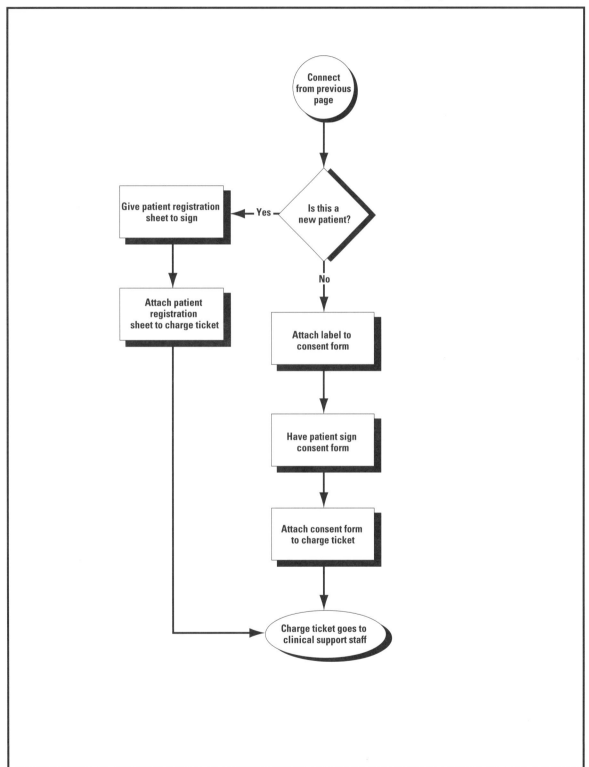

Figure 6

New Documentation and Posting Process

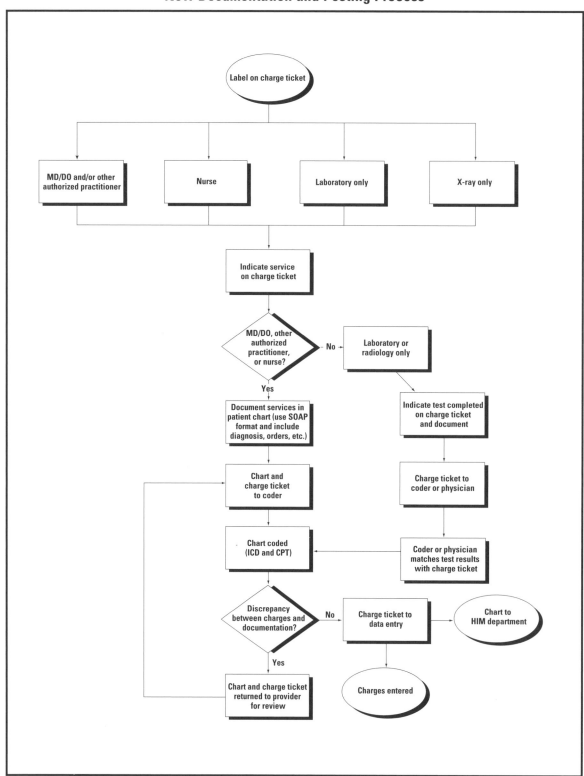

With one success under its belt, Fairview Clinics is not resting on its laurels. A new CQI initiative is currently underway—to assess reimbursement and denial trends and determine if they reveal additional possibilities for improving documentation and posting. Wieland says Fairview is now committed to reviewing all its processes and systems continuously.

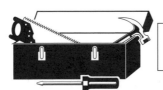

TOOLS: brainstorming, surveys, flow charts, PDCA method

Vital Statistics

Organization: Harris Methodist Fort Worth

Type: Acute Care

Location: Fort Worth, Texas

Size: 628 beds

Caseload: 26,400 inpatients and 40,000 outpatient and emergency visits per year

Affiliation: Texas Health Resources (16 hospitals, as well as long-term care, assisted-living, and skilled-nursing facilities)

Making the Most of Databases and Registries

Healthcare organizations spend a lot of time collecting data—so much, in fact, that they may have little time available for effective analysis. Furthermore, reliance on chart review as a data-collection tool can generate a mountain of chart requests for HIM staff to process. It's a dilemma that a CQI team at this Texas hospital decided to address.

Overview

Like most healthcare organizations, Harris Methodist Hospital in Fort Worth, Texas, maintains a variety of database administrators and registries to monitor treatment trends, patient outcomes, and quality indicators. As staff in the hospital's health information services (HIS) department process and complete patient records, they collect much of the information needed to maintain these databases, so database managers and quality personnel have traditionally relied on chart review as a data-collection tool. In fact, said Larry Dunham, RRA, director of HIS at Harris Methodist, about 20-25 percent of the chart requests fielded by his department—as many as 200 chart requests per week—came from personnel who were collecting statistical information for databases. Balancing these requests with the treatment-related requests of physicians, while also expediting chart completion and billing, was a heavy burden.

Reliance on patient charts was not always convenient for database administrators, though. The widespread demand for data often meant administrators had to wait their turn to review a chart, making data-collection frustrating and time-consuming. Indeed, said Dunham, the organization tended to spend so much time collecting data, staff had little time for the kind of analysis needed to generate concrete improvement initiatives. Computerizing patient records would improve accessibility and help make the collection process more efficient, but, as in many facilities, the transition to an electronic record at Harris Methodist will be a slow, complex process.

Nonetheless, Dunham felt there had to be opportunities for streamlining data collection, using, among other things, other electronic sources. The HIS department, he knew, maintains its own data-abstract database, known as Code 3, which tracks most of the information stored in patient charts—including patient demographics, diagnoses, and procedures. Encouraging and enabling on-line data collection through Code 3, instead of via paper records, might, Dunham speculated, ease the chart-request burden on HIS staff and reduce the time needed for data-collection. This, in turn, would allow database administrators to spend more time putting organizational data to constructive use. In 1996, Dunham and the director of continuous improvement assembled a 10-person quality-improvement team to explore this and other possibilities for improving data-collection and Harris Methodist's use of databases.

Getting started

Harris Methodist's institutionalized CQI method is a five-step adaptation of the PDCA approach (Plan, Do, Check, Act), known as the VALUE method (see Figure 1).

CQI teams are guided through each step by a team leader and a facilitator, who assume complementary leadership roles. The team leader takes responsibility for the day-to-day mechanics of the process and the ultimate outcome. The facilitator maintains a broader perspective—monitoring the team's overall goals, coaching the team leader, and stepping in if the team members seem to be straying too far off track.

In this instance, Dunham served as team leader; he organized and ran team meetings, documented the team's progress, and assessed its work at each stage. Margaret Proctor, RRA, CPHQ, director of continuous improvement, served as facilitator. She worked closely with Dunham throughout the initiative; at meetings she was expected to listen, ask constructive and leading questions, and intervene if members seemed to be losing focus. The other team members included a representative from information

Figure 1

VALUE Method

	STEP	OBJECTIVE
V	**VALIDATE problems/opportunities**	Identify and define an area or process for improvement based on customer requirements and data
A	**ANALYZE the process**	Identify and verify reasons ("root causes") that underlie problems or that create opportunities for improvement
L	**LIST improvements**	Propose and evaluate steps for improvement and plan their implementation
U	**USE improvements**	Get approval for planned improvements and implement them
E	**EVALUATE results**	Assess the effectiveness of improvements and ensure their standardization and replication

Compiled with permission from: Harris Methodist: Continuous Improvement Handbook (©1994 Harris Methodist and Total Quality Management Services, Inc.), which includes material adapted from Avatar International, Inc.

technology, an HIS staff member who was familiar with the Code 3 database, and individuals involved in the largest and most active of Harris Methodist's other registries and databases. (Note: The CQI initiative examined the operations and activities of 14 internal databases, but not all of them were represented on the team.)

At its first meeting, Dunham introduced the team's main objective: to build an efficient system of data retrieval, storage, analysis, and reporting. Then he outlined a number of goals designed to help the team achieve that objective (see Figure 2).

Analysis: Identifying problems

Once Dunham had outlined the team's mission, team members held brainstorming sessions that identified six opportunity areas (see Figure 3a).

Figure 2

CQI Objective and Goals

OBJECTIVE:
Build an efficient system of data retrieval, storage, analysis, and reporting

GOALS:
1. Streamline data collection and data entry processes
   - Identify and eliminate redundancies
   - Eliminate unnecessary collection
2. Establish lines of communication between databases
3. Standardize data capture and reporting procedures
4. Enable collection of data while it's timely and useful

Six areas seemed like a lot to tackle, so team members set out to prioritize them. They established four criteria for evaluating the opportunity areas: 1) impact on quality; 2) cost-effectiveness; 3) ease of implementation; and 4) ability to pilot (i.e., to perform a small-scale trial run). Then they used a decision matrix to rank each area according to

Figure 3a

Opportunities for Improvement

1. **Fewer reviews:** decrease need for chart reviews by facilitating reliance on HIS electronic database
2. **Share information:** increase sharing of data between databases to eliminate redundant collection
3. **Idle moments:** facilitate chart reviews during idle periods of chart completion (before filing) to reduce time spent pulling filed charts
4. **Data integrity:** improve integrity of data gathered by facilitating reliance on HIS electronic database
5. **Opportunistic collection:** identify other (non-HIS) sources of on-line data to reduce reliance on chart review
6. **Strategic collection:** audit data that's gathered to eliminate unnecessary collection

how well it met the goals and intent of those criteria (see Figure 3b, pages 124–125). The areas that received the highest priority rankings tended to be those that involved assessing the type of data being collected and streamlining collection methods, so the team chose to focus its analysis on those areas.

To facilitate its analysis, the team sought to develop a better understanding of how the databases operated. What information did each database administrator collect? Why? Where did it come from? What were their collection triggers (that is, how did they isolate relevant patients and cases)? The administrators for each of the 14 databases under examination were asked to submit the forms or tools they used to abstract patient information for entry into their databases. Then each administrator was asked to explain how they gathered that information and to develop a flow chart illustrating their process (see Figures 4a & 4b, pages 126–127). By comparing the information that each database administrator provided, team members noticed redundancies and began to identify data that was available via sources other than the patient record.

Listing opportunities and proposing solutions

According to Dunham, the most obvious redundancy involved collection of basic patient-demographic information, which each database needed. The data was available in the Code 3 database and in the hospital mainframe system, but the other database administrators were still abstracting it from paper-based patient records. A number of the administrators simply didn't know patient demographics were available on-line, while security procedures prevented some from accessing Code 3 and mainframe data. Educating database administrators about Code 3 and mainframe content, and updating security procedures to improve their access, seemed likely to streamline this component of data collection.

In addition, the review of data-collection procedures revealed that the infection control database could draw clinical data from Code 3, as well as demographics data. The infection control registry tracks infection diagnoses in the patient population to help the hospital identify at-risk patients and design procedures for preventing infection. Since Code 3 tracks the diagnoses and procedures data that this database needs, there was no need for the infection-control administrator to be reviewing charts. Helping her shift to an on-line mode of collection, says Dunham, dramatically reduced the amount of time that she spent on collection and virtually eliminated a source of chart requests.

Figure 3b

Decision Matrix

	CRITERIA					
OPPORTUNITY AREAS	Quality Impact weight: 4	Cost Effectiveness weight: 5	Ease of Implementation weight: 5	Ability to Pilot weight: 5	Weighted-Score Total	Rank
Fewer Reviews	2 / 8	3 / 15	2 / 10	3 / 15	48	3
Share Information	1 / 4	3 / 15	1 / 5	2 / 10	34	5
Idle Moments	1 / 4	3 / 15	2 / 10	3 / 15	44	4
Data Integrity	3 / 12	3 / 15	2 / 10	3 / 15	52	2
Opportunistic Collection	2 / 8	3 / 15	3 / 15	3 / 15	53	1
Strategic Collection	3 / 12	3 / 15	2 / 10	3 / 15	52	2

Scoring	Weighting
How well does this opportunity area meet the goal of this criterion?	How important is this criterion relative to the others?
1 = poorly 2 = adequately 3 = well	3 = unimportant 4 = important 5 = very important
note scores to the left of the diagonals dividing the score boxes	*weighted score to the right of the diagonal = score multiplied by criterion weight*

Deciphering the matrix

As discussed in Chapter 4, "CQI Tools," a decision matrix is useful for objectively comparing and analyzing data in order to rank findings and set priorities. This matrix compares six opportunity areas, which are listed on the left-hand side. Criteria for evaluating those opportunity areas are listed along the top.

The "weight" noted in each criterion box ranks that criterion's importance. Weighting ensures that more important criteria have a greater influence on the overall priority rating; in this case, "impact on quality" has slightly less influence on the final priority rankings than the other criteria.

To establish priorities, the six opportunity areas are scored according to how well they fulfill the goals or intent of each criterion. Those scores are entered on the left side of the boxes that are divided diagonally (1 = poor; 2 = adequate; 3 = well). The scores are then multiplied by the weight for each respective criterion, and the product, or weighted score, is entered to the right of the diagonal line. The weighted scores are totaled to determine the relative value of each opportunity area. The opportunity area with the highest weighted score becomes the top priority.

While other databases—the tumor registry and the open-heart surgery registry, for instance—also needed the information on diagnoses and procedures in Code 3 and the mainframe, their administrators did track some data that the HIS database could not provide. In these instances, the CQI team focused its efforts in two areas: First, it tried to identify opportunities for information sharing—instances, that is, in which databases were collecting the same information. For example, the birth registry and the neonatal intensive care registry each tracked birth-weight data; yet the database administrators for each had always collected that data separately: two people, two chart requests, one piece of information. Linking the databases and centralizing entry of birth-weight data, therefore, seemed likely to make both databases a bit more efficient and to reduce the number of chart requests submitted by those administrators.

Figure 4a

Trauma Registry: Data-Identification Process

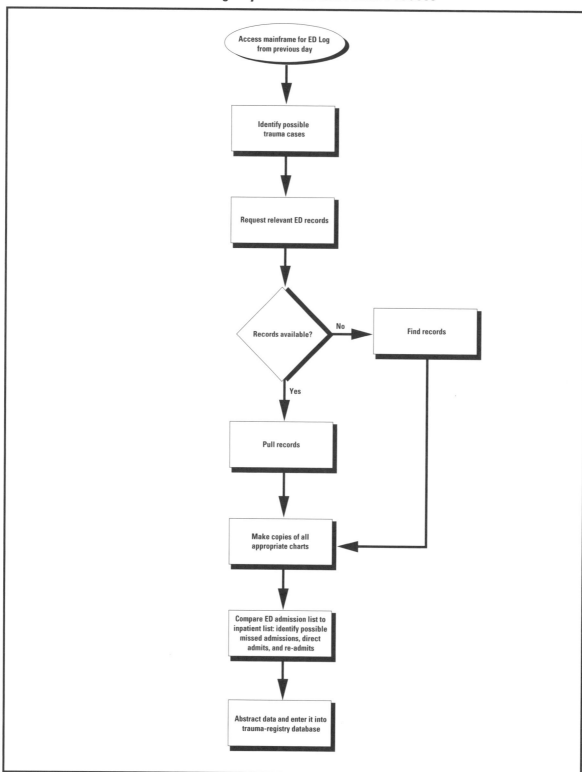

Figure 4b

Tumor Registry: Data-Identification Process

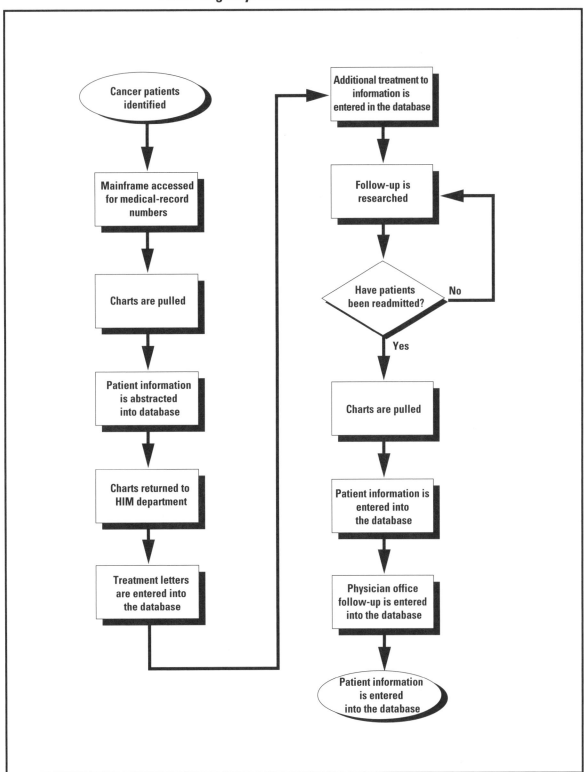

The CQI team was not satisfied simply to identify opportunities for information sharing and reduce the number of redundant chart requests, however. As much as possible, team members wanted to eliminate chart review as a data-collection tool, which meant they had to identify alternative tools. Team members knew, for instance, that the pharmacy's medication records tracked patient weight, so they established procedures that allowed the birth and neonatal registries to avoid chart reviews by accessing the birth-weight information stored in the pharmacy's computers. Pharmacy computers also became a valuable source of information for databases that tracked medication orders. Surprisingly enough, so did accounts-receivable files; in fact, by accessing billing records, the CQI team found that database administrators could gather a wide range of treatment- and service-related information, including data on medication use. The team also created interfaces with lab computers for databases that monitored test-result data. These interfaces reduced, for example, the tumor registry's reliance on chart reviews for information from pathology reports.

Did it work?

Change is unsettling and, in some cases, the team reengineered database operations in significant ways. But Dunham said that, before long, the database administrators were embracing new procedures that, as he'd hoped, were reducing the amount of time needed for data collection and increasing the time available for analyzing data and using it to improve processes and patient outcomes. Meanwhile, according to Dunham, database-related chart requests are down about 33 percent in the HIS department, fewer doctors are complaining about chart availability, and the HIS staff has more time to work on chart completion. Modern healthcare organizations collect all kinds of data, said Dunham, but they often do a bad job of communicating about what they're collecting and where it's stored. Key to the success of Harris Methodist's CQI effort, he said, was the team's ability to take an honest, comprehensive look at the data that the hospital collected and to find creative ways for accessing that data and putting it to use.

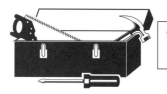

TOOLS: brainstorming, surveys/interviews, decision matrix, flow charts, adapted PDCA method

Vital Statistics

Organization: Morton Plant Mease Health Care

Type: Integrated Delivery System

Location: Tampa Bay-area, Florida

Facilities: 4 hospitals (1,217 beds); 3 ambulatory-care centers; 1 physician health organization; wellness and community-care centers

CQI Averts Delinquent-Records Crisis

Taking a proactive approach to CQI often allows organizations to spot and correct problems in their earliest stages—before they become damaging crises. A case in point is this Florida-based hospital network that nipped a delinquent-records trend in the bud.

Overview

Alarm bells don't literally start clanging when something is out of whack at Florida-based Morton Plant Mease Health Care (MPM). But you'd almost think they do, given the speed with which the Tampa Bay-area organization launches improvement initiatives. For instance, in January 1997, the number of delinquent records spiked above 1,200 across MPM's three hospital campuses (Morton Plant Mease has since acquired a fourth hospital). That total was well below the approximately 1,600 delinquencies that the JCAHO permits in a hospital network MPM's size (then about 1,100 beds and 3,115 discharges per month), but it was 50 percent above the HIM department's internal standard of 800 delinquencies. The HIM department assembled a CQI task force to evaluate the increase in delinquencies and to recommend improvements. By July, the delinquency rate dropped below 700 and stayed there.

The buck stops in HIM

Patient charts are not considered complete or legally valid until physicians have dictated and signed certain documents. Because information in the chart is crucial to quality of care, the Joint Commission on Accreditation of Healthcare Organizations (JCAHO) gives doctors 30 days to sign those documents. Morton Plant Mease seeks to protect its JCAHO accreditation status by suspending the admitting privileges of doctors who fail to sign within 28 days.

Nonetheless, MPM's 15-person CQI team—comprised entirely of HIM employees—chose not to address the organization's delinquency problem by applying additional pressure to physicians. MPM's HIM department, like many others, views the medical staff as a key customer and CQI team members felt it would be counter-productive to apply more pressure to doctors. The team felt that doctors would be more likely to cooperate with CQI initiatives if they viewed the HIM department as an ally. Besides, CQI team members felt that they should focus on finding opportunities to improve HIM processes—in large part because the HIM department controls access to most charts needing signatures.

With those parameters in mind, the team set three goals for their initiative: 1) Work with physicians to decrease the number of delinquent charts. 2) Increase physician satisfaction with HIM. 3) Decrease the number of chart-analysis errors.

Bar-coding system and statistical indicators drive CQI

Electronic data collection powers Morton Plant Mease's CQI process. The organization's computers continuously capture data on HIM functions. That information is updated regularly—in some cases, concurrently—so up-to-the-minute quality assessment is possible.

An innovative bar-coding system is one of the key components of this electronic data collection. MPM initially installed the system to track chart location and to expedite fulfillment of chart requests. However, bar coding also allows for instantaneous data collection and reporting.

The bar-coding system is a useful tool for tracking key delinquent-records indicators because, in addition to telling where a chart is, it also tells HIM employees how long the chart has been there. When a patient is discharged, for instance, the chart goes first through inpatient assembly and analysis (IAA) and coding, where the respective staffs have a total of three days to place the materials in universal chart order, to check the contents and documentation, to note what materials a physician still needs to dictate, to flag reports that need a physician's signature, and to input diagnosis and procedure codes. When that process is complete, the chart goes to the physicians' workroom, where doctors dictate and/or sign reports. Once charts are signed and complete, they go into the permanent files. When the chart arrives in both IAA and coding, the bar code is swiped. When it arrives in the workroom, it's swiped again. At that point, the computer notes whether the HIM staff met the three-day deadline for IAA and coding and it begins the countdown for physicians. When charts are signed and ready for permanent filing, the bar code is swiped once more and the computer notes how many days have passed since discharge. If the entire process—from discharge to permanent filing—takes more than 28 days, the system registers that chart as delinquent and the HIM department suspends the physician in question.

The bar-coding system, therefore, provided three of the five key indicators that MPM identified as having triggered the CQI initiative on delinquencies and customer service (see Figure 1, Indicators 1, 2, and 4)—that is, it allowed HIM to track: 1) the number of delinquent charts, 2) the number of days it took to sign charts, and, 3) the number of days it took for assembly, analysis, and coding. The other two key indicators for the CQI team included physician suspensions and analysis errors, which HIM also monitors electronically.

Figure 1

Key Indicators

1. Number of delinquent charts
2. Average number of days taken to sign
3. Number of physicians on suspension
4. Time spent on chart assembly and analysis
5. Number of analysis errors

Identifying problems, proposing solutions

Armed with this initial indicator data, the CQI team held brainstorming sessions to identify likely problem areas and opportunities for improvement. In keeping with its goals, the team emphasized ideas for improving processes and performance within

HIM, hoping this would promote a spirit of cooperation and would produce better results than strategies and tactics geared toward pressuring doctors to "do better."

Following is a sampling of problems the team identified, and solutions it proposed:

Inconsistent policies and procedures

Even though the HIM department was integrated across all three MPM hospital campuses, the policies governing chart analysis were not; one hospital's was different.

Solution: The CQI team decided that drafting a standard policy would lessen physician and analyzer confusion, help reduce the number of analysis errors, and begin to limit delays due to rework.

Poor quality control

HIM had few, if any, mechanisms for catching analysis errors before charts reached physicians. This was damaging from a physician-satisfaction standpoint because the doctors often spotted mistakes before HIM. Furthermore, the delays involved in correcting errors and resubmitting the charts for signing affected the chart-completion and delinquency rates.

Solution: HIM began auditing the results of chart analysis to catch errors earlier and to identify training needs within the department.

Who's the attending?

The analysis audits, as well as input from physicians, revealed that analyzers sometimes assigned charts to the wrong attending physician—especially if the attending physician had been changed mid-treatment, or if the patient had seen several doctors. Delays while the chart made its way to the right doctor affected completion time and the delinquency rate.

Solution: The CQI team developed and distributed a flow chart that outlines the process for making the attending-physician designation, and that tells analyzers where to go for help when designation information is not immediately apparent (see Figure 2).

Figure 2

Process for Designating Attending Physician

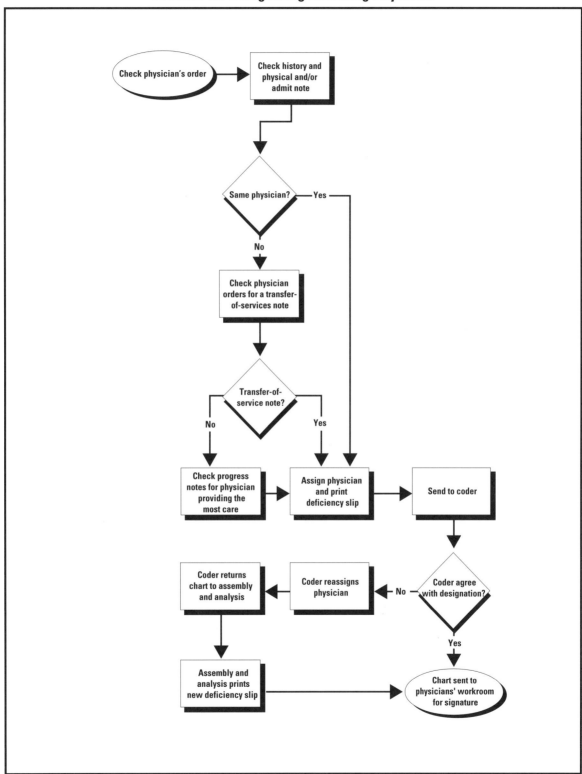

Bad bar coding

Employees are supposed to swipe the bar code as soon as a chart changes locations, otherwise tracking and data collection are inaccurate. For instance, a chart that isn't swiped when it arrives in the permanent files will eventually appear on the delinquent list because the computer still assumes it is unsigned. The team theorized that unreliable use of the bar-coding system might be inflating the delinquency rate and prompting undeserved suspensions.

> **Solution:** The CQI team held bar-coding audits to identify errors and lapses and gave staff a refresher course on using the system properly.

Physicians on the move

Because physicians often see patients at different MPM campuses and in their own practices, their schedules are unpredictable. The team realized that doctors sometimes go days, or even weeks, without visiting a particular hospital, which means their charts sit unsigned at that campus.

> **Solution:** The HIM department enhanced its efforts to alert doctors of approaching signing deadlines. And, at a doctor's request, or if a deadline was imminent, the team began sending documents to other locations for signing. The team also recommended delivering charts to doctors who were on-campus but too busy to get to the physicians' workroom.

Vacations

HIM is not supposed to suspend a doctor who is on vacation, provided none of the doctor's charts are delinquent when the doctor leaves. Nor, however, are doctors supposed to leave without signing charts that are delinquent. Since HIM rarely knew physician vacation schedules, staff tended to count vacation days against physicians and often weren't able to encourage doctors to make time for signing before taking time off.

> **Solution:** The CQI team worked with medical staff personnel to establish mechanisms for communicating physician vacation schedules to HIM.

Us vs. them

There was not enough communication between physicians and HIM staff on issues regarding chart delinquencies. This meant there were few opportunities to share ideas and celebrate successes.

Solution #1: The CQI team developed a survey (see Figure 3) that captured physician input on the chart-signing/completion process.

Solution #2: The CQI team arranged to have HIM hold periodic celebrations for physicians who signed their charts on time.

Figure 3

Physician Survey

WHAT CAN THE WORKROOM TEAM DO TO IMPROVE THE CHART-COMPLETION PROCESS?

_____

_____

_____

_____

_____

_____

**PLEASE PLACE YOUR COMPLETED SURVEY IN THE
BOX IN THE PHYSICIANS' WORKROOM**

Results and follow-up

Morton Plant Mease's electronic data-collection tools allowed the CQI team to monitor the results of its improvement initiatives. Using that data, the team developed a run chart that illustrates how dramatically chart delinquencies decreased (see Figure 4). The delinquency rate hovered above MPM's internal standard of 800 charts per month (half the total allowed by the JCAHO) through June. But it dipped to 690 in July, and did not top 700 again.

For the most part, the physician suspension rate also dropped off significantly. The total number of suspensions peaked above the January level of 304 twice, but hovered closer to 200 for all but two months after June (see Figure 5). At the end of the year, HIM scored an 89-percent approval rating from physicians on an annual MPM survey that gauges the performance of all departments.

Results of the team's efforts to reduce analysis errors were mixed. Changing documentation requirements kept the team from standardizing assembly and analysis procedures until early 1998; in all but one month of 1997 (April), there were more analysis errors than there had been in January (16). The error rate peaked at triple the January level in May (48), and closed the year up about 50 percent compared to January (see Figure 6). Because the actual number of errors was relatively small, though—often only a dozen or two—a small change tended to produce dramatic and somewhat

Figure 4

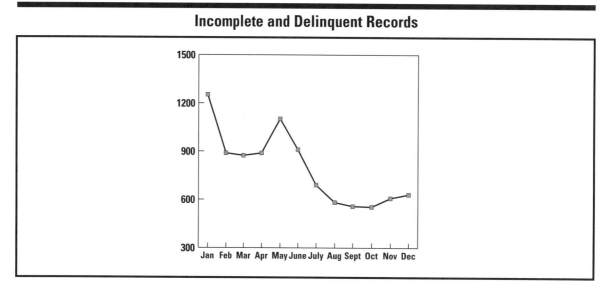

Incomplete and Delinquent Records

Figure 5

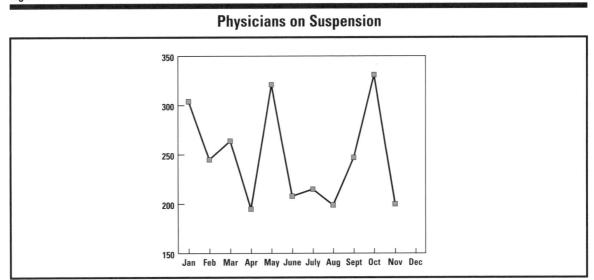

Physicians on Suspension

Figure 6

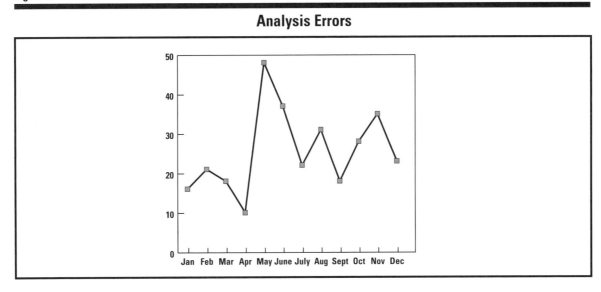

Analysis Errors

deceiving run-chart fluctuations. Nonetheless, team members plan to continue monitoring error rates and seeking additional opportunities to improve procedures and performance.

Special thanks to Pamela Haines, RRA—former manager of operations at Morton Plant Mease Health Care, and now director of medical records at Operation PAR, Inc.—for her help with this case study.

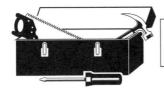

Tools: Brainstorming, Survey, Flow Chart, Run Charts, PDCA Method

Vital Statistics

Organization: Roper Home Care Services

Type: Hospital-affiliated home-care agency

Location: Charleston, South Carolina

Caseload: Approximately 90,000 home-care visits per year

Home Care Agency Tackles Late and Unsigned Orders

It is, perhaps, the most difficult accreditation requirement for home-care agencies to meet: ensuring that doctors sign orders and plans of care within the timeframe set by the state and the JCAHO. Thanks to a committed CQI team, this South Carolina agency saw its on-time return rate increase eight-fold in a single year.

by Deborah Hepburn, RN, MS

Overview

In fall 1995, Medicare began investigating an increase in billing for physical-therapy visits by Roper Home Care Services (RHCS), a hospital-affiliated home-care agency located in Charleston, South Carolina. Investigators asked to review 100 to 200 charts per month and, in an effort to correct inadvertent billing mistakes before submission, Roper's four-person HIM staff audited the documentation and billing information in those charts.

Recognizing the valuable effect these audits were having on data integrity and billing accuracy, the staff expanded them to cover all records. As a result, they began to realize that Roper had significant problems getting physicians to sign orders and plans of care—also known as 485s. As of April 1996, doctors were signing barely one in ten (about 11 percent) of Roper's 485s within 30 days, as required by the Joint Commission on Accreditation of Healthcare Organizations (JCAHO). In fact, almost half (47 percent) of the plans of care that Roper sent out for signature were never returned. Technically, therefore, RHCS was providing a great deal of care without proper legal authorization, and nearly half of the agency's Medicare billing was not properly documented and at risk of being denied. Concerned, RHCS launched a CQI initiative. By April 1997, doctors were signing 90 percent of the 485s on time, and the overall return rate soared to 99.7 percent (including plans of care that were signed late).

The plan-of-care dilemma

The Home Health Certification and Plan of Care, or 485, is a standard form that doctors must sign to authorize an order for home-care services for a Medicare patient (see Figure 1). Home-care providers often use the 485 format to certify non-Medicare patients, too. Current (1998) JCAHO home-care standards require agencies to have a signed plan of care in a patient's record no more than 30 days after an order is issued, and in less time if state regulations so require. By 1999, JCAHO is expected to lift its 30-day requirement, meaning surveyors will note only whether home-care facilities comply with existing state laws and regulations. The commission is also expected to stop punishing agencies when physicians sign orders late, provided the fault lies with the doctor (that is, provided the agency has adequate procedures in place for securing signatures and can demonstrate that it made a concerted effort to obtain missing or late signatures in the time allotted). With or without these changes, however, home-care facilities still need procedures for ensuring that doctors sign plans of care and other orders in a timely fashion.

Hospitals and other organizations face similar requirements, but obtaining signatures can be particularly problematic for home-care providers—in large part because the setting is so decentralized. Doctors who order home-care services don't work at the agencies that provide the services; there's no opportunity for HIM staff to stop physicians in the hall, and there are few avenues for holding special promotions or campaigns to remind physicians to sign. Furthermore, as the number of home-care agencies increases, doctors have more referral options. Pursuing signatures too aggressively may discourage future referrals and hurt an agency's bottom line. In short, the CQI team at RHCS had to weigh its options carefully as it considered how to respond to its delinquency problem.

Nonetheless, the agency knew it had to respond; 485s are too important. Without signed plans of care, clinical staff at RHCS cannot legally care for patients, Medicare can deny payment for services performed, and patient records are not considered

Figure 1

Sample Plan of Care

Department of Health and Human Services Health Care Financing Administration	Form Approved OMB No. 098-0357

HOME HEALTH CERTIFICATION AND PLAN OF CARE

1. Patient's HI Claim No.	2. Start of Care Date	3. Certification Period From: To:	4. Medical Record No.	5. Provider No.

6. Patient's Name and Address	7. Provider's Name, Address, and Telephone Number

8. Date of Birth	9. Sex ❏ M ❏ F	10. Medications: Dose / Frequency /Route (N)ew (C)hanged

11. ICD-9-CM	Principal Diagnosis	Date
12. ICD-9-CM	Surgical Procedure	Date
13. ICD-9-CM	Other Pertinent Diagnoses	Date

14. DME and Supplies	15. Safety Measures
16. Nutritional Req.	17. Allergies

18.A. Functional Limitations
1 ❏ Amputation
2 ❏ Bowel/Bladder (Incontinence)
3 ❏ Contracture
4 ❏ Hearing
5 ❏ Paralysis
6 ❏ Endurance
7 ❏ Ambulation
8 ❏ Speech
9 ❏ Legally Blind
A ❏ Dyspnea with Minimal Exertion
B ❏ Other (Specify)

18.B. Activities Permitted
1 ❏ Complete Bedrest
2 ❏ Bedrest BRP
3 ❏ Up As Tolerated
4 ❏ Transfer Bed/Chair
5 ❏ Exercises Prescribed
6 ❏ Partial Weight Bearing
7 ❏ Independent At Home
8 ❏ Crutches
9 ❏ Cane
A ❏ Wheelchair
B ❏ Walker
C ❏ No Restrictions
D ❏ Other (Specify)

19. Mental Status
1 ❏ Oriented
2 ❏ Comatose
3 ❏ Forgetful
4 ❏ Depressed
5 ❏ Disoriented
6 ❏ Lethargic
7 ❏ Agitated
8 ❏ Other

20. Prognosis
1 ❏ Poor
2 ❏ Guarded
3 ❏ Fair
4 ❏ Good
5 ❏ Excellent

21. Orders for Discipline and Treatments (Specify Amount/Frequency/Duration)

22. Goals/Rehabilitation Potential/Discharge Plans

23. Nurse's Signature and Date of Verbal SOC Where Applicable:	25. Date HHA Received Signed POT

24. Physician's Name and Address	26. I certify/recertify that this patient is confined to his/her home and needs intermittent skilled nursing care, physical therapy and/or speech therapy or continues to need occupational therapy. The patient is under my care, and I have authorized the services on this plan of care and will periodically review the plan.
27. Attending Physician's Signature and Date Signed	28. Anyone who misrepresents, falsifies, or conceals essential information required for payment of Federal funds may be subject to fine, imprisonment, or civil penalty under applicable Federal laws.

Form HCFA–485 (C–3) (02–94) (Print Aligned)

complete and valid. The retrospective audits that had uncovered the delinquent- and missing-signature problem were OK as a temporary method for flagging unsigned documents, but they required the full-time attention of three of the agency's four HIM employees and could not, therefore, continue indefinitely. RHCS needed an effective and lower-maintenance solution.

Putting CQI to work

RHCS employs an adaptation of the PDCA method for CQI known as FOCUS PDCA (see Figure 2). As the acronym suggests, the five steps in the FOCUS phase are designed to guide preliminary analysis to help ensure development of effective, targeted improvement initiatives. This preliminary analysis might normally be included in the planning (P) phase of the traditional PDCA approach. The five

Figure 2

FOCUS PDCA Method

F	FIND a process to improve	Define the problem(s) Identify affected customers
O	ORGANIZE to make improvements	Define effects on customers Establish mission of CQI team Set timeframe for CQI process
C	CLARIFY knowledge of problem(s)	Analyze problem(s) Set goals for achieving CQI mission
U	UNDERSTAND root causes	Identify reasons (root causes) for problem(s) Brainstorm solutions
S	SELECT feasible solution(s)	Evaluate proposed solutions Accept the best Seek approval for implementation
P	PLAN implementation of solution(s)	Write an action plan
D	DO the implementation	Implement action-plan tactics
C	CHECK the results	Monitor and evaluate results
A	ACT on evaluation of results	Revise and/or standardize new policies and procedures Address new or related issues as needed

FOCUS stages, however, separate the preliminary analysis needed to identify improvement initiatives from the activities involved in implementing those initiatives.

After defining the problem and organizing themselves to address it, RHCS's interdisciplinary CQI team—which included representatives from finance, the clinical staff, purchasing, HIM, and the performance improvement department—held a brainstorming session to identify factors that could be contributing to the physician-signature problem. The resulting list of 28 problems was overwhelmingly long. But further analysis revealed that the 28 problems tended to fall under six broad categories, so the team created a cause-and-effect diagram (sometimes called a fishbone diagram) that broke the large list into a series of more manageable assignment areas (see Figure 3).

Identifying problems that contributed to plan-of-care delinquencies helped shift the CQI team's outlook in an important and constructive direction. As RHCS became aware of the delinquency problem, it was not uncommon for staff to place all the blame on doctors. "Why don't they just sign?" staff would ask. But the CQI team's preliminary analysis showed that, in fact, the issue was more complex; agency staff were overlooking potentially significant problems associated with their procedures for processing 485s, and team members realized that they couldn't just focus on pressuring doctors to sign. They also needed to examine internal HIM processes and take steps to encourage physicians to cooperate with the agency.

Maximizing the team's efficiency and reach

During two one-hour sessions, the CQI team completed its cause-and-effect diagram and assigned a team member to oversee development of improvement initiatives for each of the categories identified. At this point, to maximize the efficiency of its efforts, the team shifted its emphasis away from formal meetings and agreed to gather, as a group, every two months. As team members talked with the people involved in each stage of order processing—from RHCS clerks and coders to physicians and physicians' staffs—email updates and informal hallway conversations kept the CQI process on track. The four-person HIM department had little time to spare for CQI and this less formal approach allowed team members to devote as much time as possible to putting ideas to work.

Figure 3

Missing Signatures: Causes and Effects

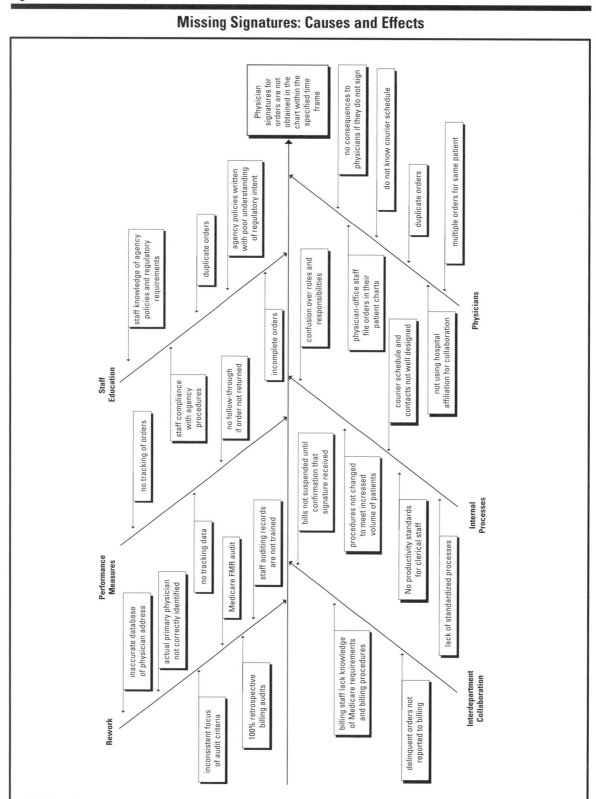

Proposing solutions

It quickly became clear that RHCS needed to formalize its procedures for generating and processing plans of care. When the organization had been small enough to store its patient records in a few milk crates, there had been little need for standard procedures. Now, however, RHCS has hundreds of active patients, and the team realized that the lack of standardization was confusing. By speaking with each person who handled plans of care and orders, the team identified key steps in the process, proposed formal procedures for handling these documents, and developed a flow chart to guide employees through the new method (see Figure 4).

In talking with field staff, team members realized that nurses were generating a lot of unnecessary orders. For instance, if a physician phoned to report a change in a patient's medication, the nurse caring for that patient often generated an order to that effect—even if RHCS would not be administering the medicine or billing for any services related to the treatment change. In other instances, nurses were writing orders based on instructions that doctors, themselves, had written on updated plans of care. (These updates, known as recertifications, are required every 62 days.) In most instances, the nurses were trying to be conscientious, but the result was a lot of unnecessary paperwork that contributed to the delinquency rate.

Interviews with physicians and their staffs, meanwhile, identified a key flaw in the way that Roper packaged and distributed 485s for signing. For some time, the agency had maintained folders for each facility with which it worked. Each week, a courier delivered a folder containing plans of care and orders for all doctors at a specific location. Staff at the medical practice distributed these documents to the appropriate physicians, and the courier returned a few days later to pick up the folder—presumably with signed orders and plans of care inside. Unfortunately, the documents did not always make their way back into the folder. Sometimes physicians misplaced them; other times office staff mistakenly filed them at the physician's office. But, whatever the reason, Roper needed a more reliable system, so the team proposed distributing doctor-specific folders. All plans of care for an individual doctor were bound inside, which meant staff at the doctor's office spent less time sorting and distributing the documents. It also meant that the 485s and orders were less likely to get lost or inadvertently filed.

Figure 4

Process for Obtaining Physician Signatures

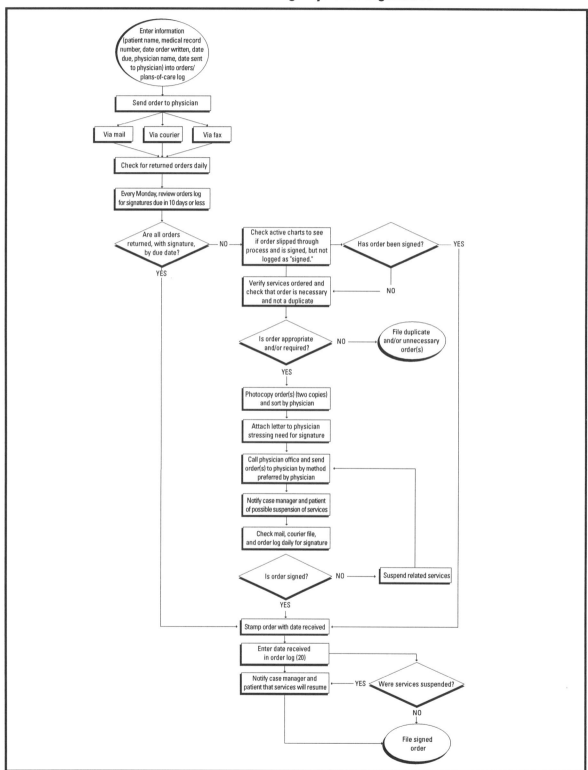

The CQI team also decided that, if all else failed, RHCS should notify doctors in writing just before orders and 485s became delinquent, warning them that the agency would be forced to discontinue the services outlined in those documents unless the doctors signed them. This was a risky proposition—first, because doctors had the option to stop referring patients to RHCS, and second, because the suspension was likely to upset patients. The team drafted a standard notification letter for doctors, which outlined the situation and explained the laws and regulations involved (see Figure 5a). To help patients better understand—and to increase pressure on physicians—the team also drafted a notification letter to be sent to patients three days before a physician's signing deadline expired (see Figure 5b). Then the team met with the medical board to discuss the implications for licensed staff and for RHCS accreditation if the delinquent- and missing-signature problem was not resolved. The board supported the notification and suspension plan, provided the agency made every attempt possible to obtain signatures up to signing deadlines, and as long as suspensions applied only to the specific services outlined in delinquent orders (all others would continue).

Monitoring results

Change can be unsettling, and, as the team introduced its improvement initiatives, some staff were resistant. Others, however, reacted positively. Some of these employees had offered suggestions in the past that were ignored; they'd begun to feel no one was listening to them or thinking about quality. Many felt they were being held responsible for problems that they could not control. Some felt they had not been given the resources and guidance they needed to succeed. These employees expressed excitement about opportunities for change; they drew energy from the CQI team's enthusiasm and demonstrated renewed commitment to their jobs.

The change initiatives produced dramatic and almost immediate results with regard to the return rate for 485s. The CQI team tracked raw data on returns in a spreadsheet log (discussed further below) and used that raw data to create run charts and bar graphs that graphically displayed the progress of their improvement efforts. While barely half the 485s and orders distributed for signature were being returned at all—late or otherwise—as of April 1996, the return rate jumped above 90 percent in May and hovered continuously near 100 percent after that (see Figure 6, page 150).

Letter to Physicians

Roper Home Care Services
Main Office
4 Carriage Lane, Suite 104
Charleston, SC 29407-1048
(803) 402-7000
Fax (803) 769-6205

Dear Dr. _____:

Please sign the enclosed orders. Occasionally, you may receive orders from months past. It is important that you sign these orders for any services we provided, even if the patient is now discharged. By Department of Health and Environmental Control (DHEC) and the Joint Commission on Accreditation of Healthcare Organizations (JCAHO) regulations, orders are to be signed and on our charts within 30 days after the order was issued. The specific regulations are stated below.*

If the orders are not received signed by the due date, our services to the patient may be discontinued. The patient will be notified of the need to suspend services until the order is signed and on the chart in the office.

We are making every effort to decrease the orders we send to you and to verify the appropriateness of the orders we request you to sign. In the past, you have received orders through the mail, facsimile, and courier. We hope that placing all orders in the folder will eliminate duplication and confusion for you and your office staff.

Our courier, Toby Stewart, will routinely visit your office to retrieve the folder and deliver current orders. Please let us know how we can better serve you and maintain compliance with the regulations. Thank you for promptly signing these orders.

Sincerely,

Director, Home Health Care

*DHEC: Reg # 61-77, Section 402 "The original plan of treatment must be signed by the patient's physician and incorporated in the record maintained by the agency for the patient. JCAHO: TX.2 & TX.2.1: "Order is obtained from the physician within the time frame...not to exceed 30 days. All Medicare-covered services are furnished under a plan of care established by a physician, and the plan of care is established before services are furnished." (An organization may accept a facsimile.)

Figure 5b

Letter to Patients

Roper Home Care Services
Main Office
4 Carriage Lane, Suite 104
Charleston, SC 29407-1048
(803) 402-7000
Fax (803) 769-6205

Date: _____ / _____ / _____

Dear _____,

Please note that Dr. _____ has not continued your prescription for home-health services, thus, we must discontinue our visits as of

_____.

In the event you have questions regarding the discontinuation of home-health services by Roper Home Care, please contact Dr. _____.

We have enjoyed serving you and, should your healthcare needs require home-health services again, we hope to provide our services to you again.

Sincerely,

_____
Service Line Director
Roper Home Health Services

cc: file

❑ 485, all services discontinued
❑ V.O. limited services discontinued

Figure 6

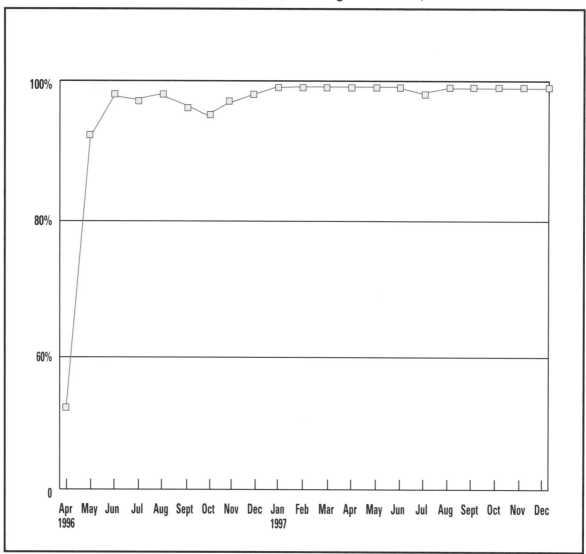

Order Return Rate (including late returns)

The percentage of orders and plans of care signed on time climbed steadily at the out-set of the CQI efforts, too. It jumped from about 11 percent in April 1996 to nearly 40 percent in May (see Figure 7). In June and July it topped 70 percent. Then, however, the tide turned. The on-time return rate began dropping steadily for four months, dipping below 60 percent again in November. From there it climbed once more, but stalled at around 80 percent in January and February of 1997. Throughout this period, the overall return rate was consistently almost 100 percent, and the team was at a loss to explain

Figure 7

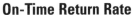

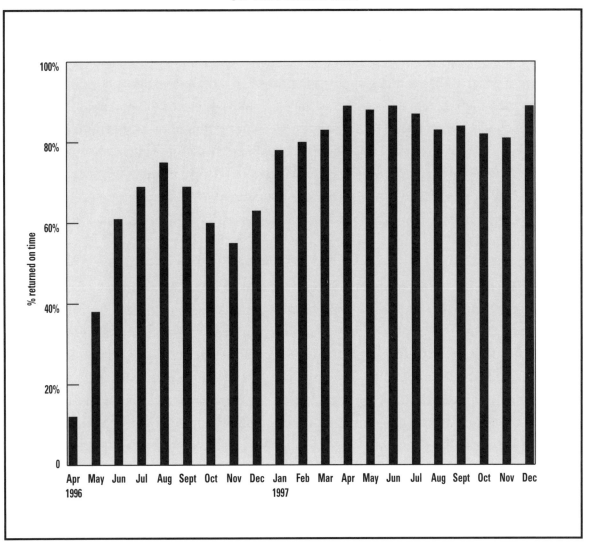

On-Time Return Rate

why, if they had such success getting orders and plans of care signed and returned, they couldn't also begin to get more of them returned within the required 30 days.

Additional interviews with RHCS field staff and referring physicians produced an unexpected explanation. Medicare required all home-care patients to be recertified every 62 days, which meant RHCS field nurses had to complete a revised plan of care with all current physician orders for the doctor to sign. For whatever reason, a good number of these recertifications were not being forwarded to doctors in a timely fashion; often they'd arrive in physician offices just a few days before the signing deadline, which made it nearly impossible for physicians to sign and return them on time. Once again, this was an example of an idiosyncratic glitch in the RHCS system that was generating delinquencies that staff might once have blamed on physicians, if they noticed it at all. Because the CQI team was monitoring the delinquency rate closely, the problem was noted quickly. More importantly, because the CQI process had created an environment in which delinquencies were being probed in a more comprehensive manner, the team identified and addressed the actual root cause of the problem. The CQI team established a mechanism for flagging all cases that required recertification ten days before the new plan of care was due. Then HIM staff began making courtesy reminder calls to field staff to complete the recertifications and submit them to physicians as efficiently as possible. Within two months (by April 1997) the on-time return rate for orders and plans of care hit 90 percent—an eight-fold increase compared to the same month a year earlier (see Figure 7).

Staff logged key information on plans of care and orders in a spreadsheet log, which tracked a wide range of information, including the patient's name, medical record number, the type of order, the physician's name, the date the order was written, the date it was sent to the physician, the date it was due in the office, and the date it was actually returned. Staff designed the program specifically to track the agency's on-time return rate, but the log also allowed them to monitor the number of orders generated each month, the time it took to generate them, the number of orders submitted to each physician, and the physicians who had the most difficulty returning signed orders as required. Throughout the CQI initiative, the log provided the team with a performance snapshot of order processing at key stages, and it fueled many of the improvement initiatives that the team generated.

Conclusion

Throughout the CQI process, each step generated more questions, more ideas, and ever-stronger support for continuous quality improvement. The order/plan-of-care issue is only one problem that RHCS has addressed during the last two years, but it provided important momentum for improvement efforts across the agency. Staff are now encouraged to give feedback, make suggestions, and participate on teams, and that encouragement has begun to produce important cultural shifts within the organization. Employees better understand how their work affects the agency as a whole, and they're less likely to feel that they'll be blamed for problems. As a result, they're more willing to identify opportunities for improvement and to take an active role in solving problems. Staff used to avoid change; now they embrace and welcome it.

As a performance improvement leader at Roper Home Care Services, Deborah Hepburn, RN, MS, launched and coordinated the CQI process that she writes about here.

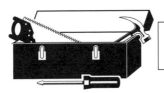

Tools: PDCA method, surveys, interviews, cause-and-effect diagram, flow charts, run charts, bar graphs.

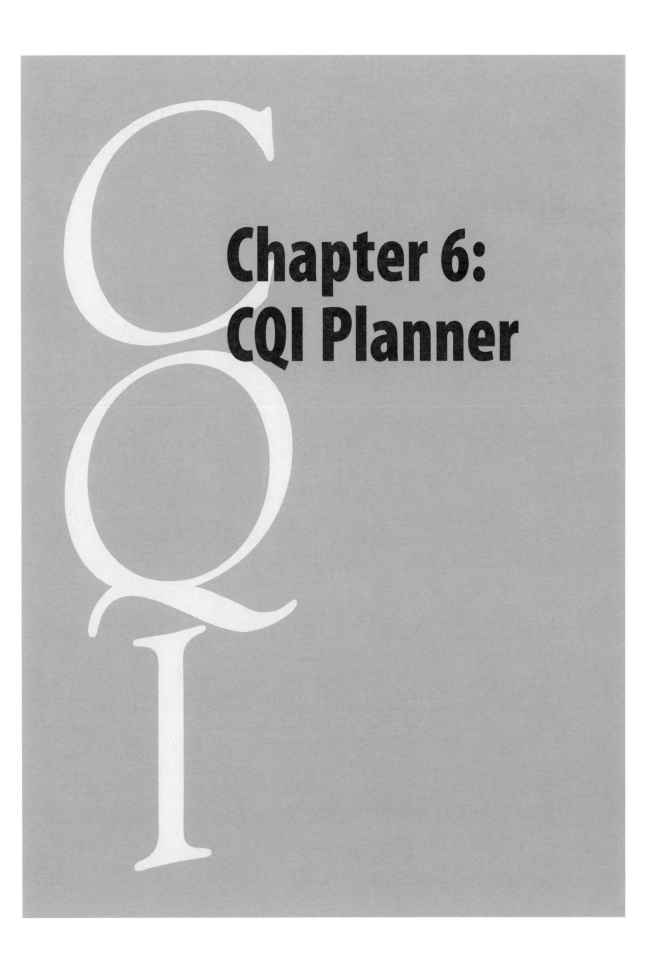

Chapter 6:
CQI Planner

Chapter 6: CQI Planner

Implementing CQI in HIM

Designing an effective CQI program and making it part of a department's culture is a challenging process. It takes determination, a willingness among managers to grant significant autonomy to staff, and a commitment from managers to help staff implement CQI techniques and overcome natural resistance to change. But the pay-off can be a department that no longer stands for below-peak performance.

Get started by immersing yourself in CQI theory. That will help you plan an approach that suits the unique needs of your department. This book is a good place to start, and its "Resource Guide" (Appendix A) lists other useful introductory materials—including works on quality, change management, and CQI by such noted authors as W. Edwards Deming, Joseph M. Juran, Philip Crosby, Mary Walton, Tom Peters, and Robert Kriegel. Familiarize yourself with the concepts in these texts and, if your continuing-education budget permits, consider attending introductory seminars on CQI.

The "CQI Planner" in this chapter is designed to be an 18-step action plan for achievement (see Figure 6.1). It outlines an 18-month, step-by-step approach to launching a CQI program in an HIM setting (Figure 6.2 provides a timeline for implementing the 18 worksteps).

You may have already completed some of the worksteps. If so, you're that much closer to establishing a department-wide CQI culture. The rest of the steps can help you see the implementation process through to the end.

If these steps won't quite mesh with unique aspects of your department, don't try to jam a square peg into a round hole. These worksteps are flexible and can serve as a jumping-off point for developing your own customized action plan and timeline.

Finally, involve managers, supervisors, and other staff in the planning process. They will be implementing and overseeing many aspects of the shift to a CQI culture, and their support for, and acceptance of, your plans will be crucial.

Figure 6.1

___

18-Step CQI Planner

Workstep #1:   Complete self-education.

Workstep #2:   Attend external CQI seminars.

Workstep #3:   Assemble and review CQI-related documents.

Workstep #4:   Meet with quality-management/assessment staff and others.

Workstep #5:   Draft a CQI plan for your department.

Workstep #6:   Update department policies and documentation.

Workstep #7:   Educate your staff.

Workstep #8:   Establish an HIM/CQI reading club.

Workstep #9:   Establish mechanisms for encouraging staff input.

Workstep #10:   Identify departmental functions, services, and products.

Workstep #11:   Identify internal and external customers.

Workstep #12:   Identify customer needs and expectations.

Workstep #13:   Establish a performance-monitoring system.

Workstep #14:   Identify and prioritize opportunities for improvement.

Workstep #15:   Establish quality-improvement teams.

Workstep #16:   Share the results of improvement projects.

Workstep #17:   Modify criteria governing employee performance evaluations.

Workstep #18:   Encourage continuous improvement.

Take it step by step

Workstep #1: Complete self-education.

As an HIM manager or director, it's up to you to get the CQI ball rolling in your department, and that means first educating yourself. The following books and videos are a good place to start (see the Appendix for a more complete list of resources):

Books:
- *The Deming Management Method*, by Mary Walton
- *Great Management Ideas from America's Most Innovative Small Companies*, by Sarah P. Noble
- *The Leadership Challenge*, by James M. Kouzes and Barry Z. Pozner
- *Kaizen: The Key to Japan's Competitive Success*, by Masaki Imai

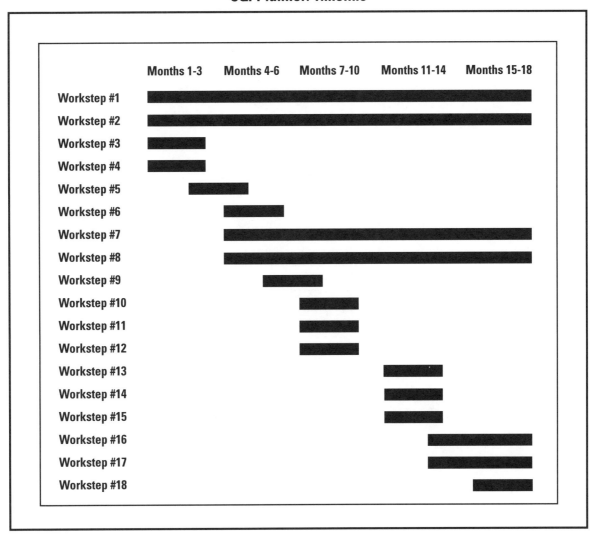

Figure 6.2

CQI Planner: Timeline

	Months 1-3	Months 4-6	Months 7-10	Months 11-14	Months 15-18
Workstep #1					
Workstep #2					
Workstep #3					
Workstep #4					
Workstep #5					
Workstep #6					
Workstep #7					
Workstep #8					
Workstep #9					
Workstep #10					
Workstep #11					
Workstep #12					
Workstep #13					
Workstep #14					
Workstep #15					
Workstep #16					
Workstep #17					
Workstep #18					

- *Unfit to Manage*, by Ernest D. Lieberman
- *The Leadership Factor*, by John P. Kotter
- *If It Ain't Broke, Break It*, by Robert Kriegel and Louis Patler
- *Sacred Cows Make the Best Burgers*, by Robert Kriegel and David Brandt
- *Thriving on Chaos*, by Thomas Peters
- *In Search of Excellence*, by Thomas Peters and Robert H. Waterman
- *Theory Why*, by John Guaspari
- *The Quality Quest*, by Wendy Leebov

Videos:

- "Quality Excellence Achieved," produced by BBP/Cally Curtis Company
- "The Business of Paradigms," produced by Charthouse Learning Corporation

Workstep #2: Attend external CQI seminars.

If departmental budgets allow, HIM management should attend two or three CQI seminars. These seminars will expose you to a range of approaches and give you an excellent base on which to build a CQI program.

Workstep #3: Assemble and review CQI-related documents.

Before outlining your CQI implementation plan, assemble and review the following documents to begin assessing how well your department is prepared for the coming changes:

- any existing quality-assessment, quality-improvement, or performance-improvement materials created by or for your department
- similar materials developed by or for other departments
- any vision statements or policies relevant to CQI, quality, performance improvement or customer service that your organization's board or other internal policy-making bodies have adopted
- CQI plans, policies, programs, and case studies that were developed by other organizations and HIM departments (internet news groups and industry magazines are a good place to look for this kind of information)
- Improvement requirements and guidelines published by accreditation and regulating agencies

Workstep #4: Meet with quality-management/assessment staff and others who can support and assist your efforts.

If possible, meet with staff that oversee quality management, quality assessment, or performance monitoring for your organization. Staff in these areas can explain hospital policies and positions that may affect development of a CQI plan for HIM. They'll also be able to offer practical support and advice as you move forward.

You should also touch base with top-level management at your organization to let them know your plans and to get their buy-in. Senior-level support will lend credibility to your efforts and help motivate your employees.

Tip: Continue to draw on these resources as you finalize and implement your CQI plan. You'll need to coordinate the changes in your department with overall hospital operations.

Workstep #5: Draft a CQI plan for your department.

Draft a CQI plan for the department that fits well with the hospital's overall policies on quality and customer service. Get input along the way from key managers and staff. If there are specific problems or opportunities that you'd like to tackle, work them into the plan. Set your goals high, but not out of sight; you don't want to so overwhelm your department with change that staff reject the culture you're trying to cultivate. Finally, develop an ambitious but realistic implementation schedule, and be prepared to adjust it as you go forward.

Workstep #6: Update department policies and documentation.

Once you've developed a CQI plan, update all policies, procedures, job descriptions, manuals, and training/orientation materials to reflect the ongoing role that CQI will play in the department. Formalizing your commitment to CQI in this way will send a powerful message to staff and help the CQI culture take root.

Workstep #7: Educate your staff.

Schedule a series of CQI inservice sessions for managers and staff. Focus on the basic concepts of CQI (see Chapter 7, "CQI Inservice Kit") and discuss key tools, techniques, and your expectations of employees. Emphasize that employees are "part owners" of the HIM department, and stress that management is committed to granting staff the autonomy and authority they'll need to drive the change process.

Use the first inservice session to introduce basic principles and the department's draft CQI plan. Tell staff what you're hoping to achieve, seek their ideas and input, and adjust your plan accordingly. The "CQI Inservice Kit" in Chapter 7 provides presentation pointers, an outline, and draft slides to help you prepare your presentation.

Keep in mind that it will take time for your staff to adjust to and accept the changes that you are proposing. Start off slowly and make sure that you and your managers talk regularly about CQI—in both formal and informal settings. Your enthusiasm and overt commitment will play an important role in securing department-wide support.

Tip: CQI education should be ongoing. Plan to send staff to "refresher" seminars periodically, continue to hold inservice sessions after the CQI program is in place, and route relevant articles and other materials around the department.

Tip: Depending on your budget, and on whether you feel comfortable training staff yourself, you might consider hiring a consultant to handle staff education. Organizations in the "Resource Guide" (Appendix A) can provide information on how to contact consultants.

Workstep #8: Establish an HIM/CQI reading club.

Book clubs have become a popular leisure-time activity for many people, and there's no reason they can't serve as the model for a professional-development program for your department. Book/reading clubs are easy to launch, inexpensive, and a good way to develop camaraderie and encourage teamwork. As you're developing a CQI program, it makes sense to have staff read books, articles, and other materials on management and quality (see Workstep #1 and the "Resource Guide" in Appendix A), but the book club could easily become a more comprehensive professional-development tool for your staff.

To launch your book club, bring staff together to discuss the concept and to pick the first book you'll all be reading. Plan to reconvene in a month or so to discuss the book. Lunch hour is a good time for the discussion meetings, since it won't interfere with the work day. End each meeting by agreeing on next month's book. To get the discussion rolling, you may want to ask a club member to open the meeting with a brief presentation.

Workstep #9: Establish mechanisms for encouraging improvement-related input from staff.

Your employees are well equipped to suggest changes; after all, they know department processes and functions inside and out. Encourage employees to contribute ideas for improving products and services by scheduling periodic brainstorming sessions and CQI-oriented "state-of-the-department" meetings. You should also post an idea board or suggestion box, and a complaints box.

Make it easy for employees to offer recommendations, and be sure to recognize and follow up on their input. In fact, as a means of empowering employees, you might want to involve the person who generated an idea in the implementation process.

Tip: Create a suggestion task force, which is made up of staff from throughout the organization who both generate ideas and solicit them from colleagues.

Tip: To encourage employees to contribute ideas, offer a prize for the "idea of the quarter."

Workstep #10: Identify departmental functions, services, and products.

As you are initiating your staff-driven CQI program, ask employees to begin the process by identifying the major functions, services, and products of your department. Several tools can facilitate this process, including: brainstorming, flow charts, surveys, and interviews (review Chapter 4, "CQI Tools," for more information).

Workstep #11: Identify internal and external customers.

A customer is anyone—from within your organization or outside it—who uses the products or services of your department. External customers include third-party payers, government agencies, etc.; internal customers include physicians, nurses, patients, billing staff, etc. Once HIM staff understand whom the department serves, they can better identify what those customers need and expect.

Workstep #12: Identify customer needs and expectations.

Once you and your staff have listed your customers, identify what those customers need and expect from your department. Internal brainstorming can help with this process, as can surveys and interviews with your customers. Surveys and interviews will also help you identify where the department's customer service is falling short. These shortcomings will undoubtedly emerge as priority action items for CQI analysis.

Workstep #13: Establish a performance monitoring system.

Ongoing performance monitoring is the key to a successful CQI program. Once you've identified your department's customers and their specific needs and expectations, you need to identify indicators that will allow you to monitor your customer service. These indicators will help you spot opportunities for improvement, and they'll identify problems before those problems become crises.

Workstep #14: Identify and prioritize opportunities for improvement.

Worksteps #11 (identifying customers) and #12 (identifying customers' needs and expectations) will give you a rough idea of where to focus your department's CQI efforts. However, it's important to prioritize improvement opportunities to keep from overwhelming staff with too many initiatives and to ensure that you tackle the most significant opportunities first. Cause-and-effect diagrams, decision matrices, and pareto charts are among the tools (discussed in Chapter 4) that can help.

Workstep #15: Establish improvement teams.

Ask employees to participate in CQI initiatives that target the high-priority opportunities that the department identified. The HIM manager or director should probably serve as team leader or facilitator, but staff should play significant, if not leading, roles. You may want to include people from outside the department on your teams. They can offer fresh perspectives on the issues being addressed. (The case studies in Chapter 5 give compelling examples of how organizations have used CQI teams.)

Workstep #16: Share the results of improvement projects.

A report summarizing the results of departmental CQI efforts is a good way to keep staff and hospital management informed about the progress of improvement initiatives. The report should profile each project underway, noting its purpose, major action steps, and results to date (see Figure 6.3). Use graphs, charts, and other CQI tools and techniques to support the report with results-oriented data. This visual evidence of improvement trends will encourage and motivate your staff, and it's an effective way to present results to senior management.

If the results of a project are particularly dramatic, submit them to your hospital's newsletter. You should also alert the public relations staff, who can begin reporting the results to external media that cover the industry. Taking these steps to share the results of CQI will help demonstrate your department's commitment to change. They will also help you recognize staff for a job well done.

Workstep #17: Modify criteria governing employee performance evaluations.

Once your CQI program is up and running, you will want to work with your managers and supervisors to create new performance-evaluation measures that are consistent with a CQI culture. Employees form the backbone of any institution, and they should be commended when they perform difficult jobs or offer ideas to improve the work

Figure 6.3

Summary Grid: CQI Results

Month Project Started	1. Project Description	2. Actions	3. Evidence of Improvement	4. Project Completed?

1. **Project purpose, objective, focus**
2. **Policy changes, work redesign, retraining/education, new equipment**
3. **Summary of what was improved**
4. **Date project completed or date of expected completion**

place. By encouraging use of CQI tools and techniques, you are also asking employees to think differently about their jobs and responsibilities; it's important that you create mechanisms for rewarding employees who rise to that challenge.

You may need to revise your evaluation system gradually, since many hospitals have long-standing guidelines and procedures that govern employee evaluations. Shifting, for instance, from quantitative standards—work or performance quotas— to qualitative guidelines for performance might be a complicated and bureaucratic process. Nonetheless, there are many ways to begin phasing in such a shift (see Figure 6.4 for a sample performance-evaluation form).

Workstep #18: Encourage continuous improvement.
Constantly remind staff to be on the lookout for improvement opportunities and

Figure 6.4

Sample Performance-Evaluation Form

Section 1: Primary Customers

Identify the three or four primary customers the associate serves and note here.

- _____   • _____
- _____   • _____

Section 2: Key Service Areas

(1) Key Service Area RESPECT: Recognizes and values the unique contribution of each team
member.

Accountabilities/Projects:

- Works cooperatively within own department and with other services.
- Willingly assumes additional responsibility to support team efforts.
- Job-specific example(s): _____

Coaching notes and results: _____

(2) Key Service Area INTEGRITY: Demonstrates integrity by adhering to the highest standards of
ethical behavior.

Accountabilities/Projects:

- Maintains confidentiality and promotes the dignity of others.
- Contributes appropriately to the changing conditions of the facility and its customers.
- Communicates with all associates in an honest and open manner.
- Job-specific example(s): _____

Coaching notes and results: _____

(3) Key Service Area SERVICE: Demonstrates commitment to service and contributes to creating
a positive, caring environment.

Accountabilities/Projects:

- Treats guests, patients, physicians, and other associates with care, courtesy, and
  respect.
- Consistently anticipates the needs of the customer and puts those needs first.
- Job-specific example(s): _____

Coaching notes and results: _____

(4) Key Service Area EXCELLENCE: Strives for excellence by building upon past accomplish-
ments and striving to achieve even higher levels of success.

Accountabilities/Projects:

- Looks for and suggests ways to continually improve our services.
- Uses past experiences as a learning process.
- Job-specific example(s): _____

Coaching notes and results: _____

Reprinted with permission of Shawnee Mission Medical Center, Shawnee Mission, Kansas.

emphasize that CQI involves constant assessment and evolution. Create forums for solciting input, and recognize contributions as a means of focusing and refocusing staff attention on CQI. Don't let enthusiasm wane.

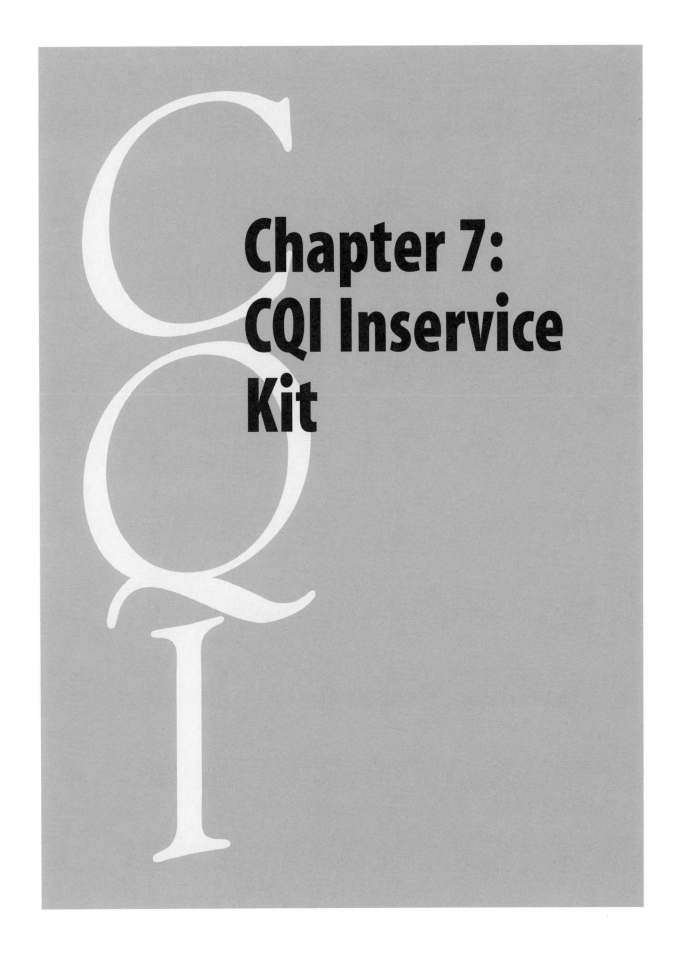

Chapter 7:
CQI Inservice Kit

Chapter 7: CQI Inservice Kit

This chapter is designed to help you generate support for CQI throughout your department and organization. It includes tips on presentations and public speaking, a suggested outline for a CQI inservice, and slides that you can use during that inservice.

Preparing for your CQI presentation

As you're thinking about your presentation, keep in mind that people absorb information in different ways: Some people like visual aids, while others prefer to listen; some people want to ask questions on the spot, while others need time to process ideas before they're ready to discuss them. It's tough to tailor a presentation that suits everyone, but slides, handouts, and reading material generally enhance your efforts. Encourage people to take notes, and leave time for questions and comments—either during or immediately after the presentation. It's also important to remain available for questions and further discussion well after the inservice is finished.

Think carefully about your objectives for the inservice to help define the length, content, and method of your presentation. If you only want to give staff an overview of CQI, a one-hour presentation on the basics is probably enough: Talk about the theories on quality and management that gave rise to continuous quality improvement in healthcare. Then address the idea of data-driven change; stress why that's so important in HIM operations and introduce some of the CQI tools that will help staff analyze departmental processes. Also emphasize the key role staff will play in the department's CQI program (the top-down support, bottom-up implementation model). Finally, discuss your plans for implementing CQI—including the timeframe you have in mind and your plans for additional staff training.

If you want to go beyond a basic introduction and begin having staff apply CQI principles—perhaps by brainstorming about department customers and their needs—you might plan a full-day session. Beef up your introductory presentation with a more in-depth explanation of the CQI tools in Chapter 4, and talk at greater length about your goals for the department and the CQI program. Don't monopolize the day, though; leave plenty of time for breakout sessions, group discussion, and Q&A.

However you design your presentation, leave yourself plenty of time to prepare. Following are a few basic "tricks of the trade" that may help:

- Know your subject
- Practice, practice, practice
- Don't rely on notes
- Use real-life examples
- Move around and encourage audience participation
- Use body language
- Be enthusiastic
- Use visual aids
- Don't rush
- Breathe and relax

Know your subject

Don't rush into presenting CQI principles to your staff before you've spent enough time on self-education. Demonstrating competence with the material will boost your credibility and make it a lot easier to transmit your goals and your enthusiasm to the whole department.

Practice, practice, practice

A lucky few of us have the ability to think through the basics of a presentation then get up in front of a group and improvise the details. The rest of us have to rehearse. Practicing ahead of time—whether it's with friends and family, with colleagues, or standing in front of the mirror—will allow you to fine tune the pacing and content of your talk. It will also help ensure that you're comfortable with the material, which allows you to focus more energy during the presentation on interacting with your audience and keeping everyone engaged.

Don't rely on notes

Use an outline or cue cards during your presentation to help you remember major points. However, try not to rely too heavily on notes, and avoid reading from a prepared text. Your natural enthusiasm and knowledge will shine through if you prepare well, create a solid framework for your presentation, then speak candidly and naturally.

Use real-life examples

During the research for your presentation, look for anecdotes that relate to CQI. That's a good way to put the material in a meaningful, real-life context for your audience. The case studies in Chapter 5 are a good place to start. Talk to others in the industry, as well, to find out how they're using improvement tools and techniques. Posting questions on internet "chat groups" is another a good way to find CQI "war stories."

Move around and encourage audience participation

If you're speaking from a podium, try not to spend the whole presentation behind it. Moving around will help settle your nerves, and it will boost your energy and enthusiasm. Ask questions when appropriate, and encourage your audience to toss out answers and provide input in other ways. Make eye contact with as many people in the audience as possible. All these tricks help keep the audience engaged, and they take some of the pressure off you.

Use body language

If you're truly excited about what you have to say, body language and gestures will happen naturally. Nonetheless, make a conscious effort to demonstrate your enthusiasm and to hammer home points by using body language effectively.

Be enthusiastic

Some people have a tendency to downplay issues during a presentation. Enthusiasm is contagious, however, and one of the best ways to get your staff excited about CQI is to demonstrate your enthusiasm for it. Try not to oversell; that can seem insincere. But in many ways underselling is worse. You want staff to leave your presentation knowledgeable, excited, and convinced of your commitment to CQI.

Use visual aids

Visual aids—slides, transparencies, videotapes, and other "props"—can help you illustrate complex points, and they help hold your audience's attention. They'll also help keep you focused and on track. (Sample slides to support a CQI presentation are included at the end of this chapter.)

Don't rush

Don't be afraid to pause, collect your thoughts, and think about where you want to go next. A few seconds of silence can seem like an eternity when you're up in front of an audience, but your listeners aren't likely to notice. In fact, a strategic pause now and then can help drive your points home. Furthermore, speaking slowly and pausing periodically will give your audience a chance to process what you're saying.

Breathe and relax

We hear it all the time: Public speaking is one of the things that people fear most. If you fall into that category, build in some time just before your presentation to relax, breathe deeply, and clear your head. Visualize yourself giving a great speech, then go out and do it.

Presentation outline

The following outline may help you prepare your CQI presentation:

CQI inservice: introductory presentation

I. Overview of CQI

(In this section, present your organization's perspective on why CQI is important.)

    A. Introduction: commitment to continuous quality improvement

    B. Why CQI is important

    C. The key players in CQI (HIM staff and other departments)

    D. Background on use of CQI in business and industry (see Chapters 2 and 3)

        1. Deming's 14 Points

        2. Introduction to the principles of Juran, Crosby, Joiner, and other quality pioneers

    E. CQI and healthcare

        1. Quality of care

        2. Expectations of accreditation and regulating agencies

II. CQI philosophy

(This section gives your staff an overview of CQI theory and addresses implementation in the context of HIM.)

    A. Why HIM needs CQI

    B. When CQI can be used in the department

    C. How the department can implement CQI

III. Major components of CQI

(This section introduces basic CQI tools and techniques.)

    A. Identifying customers and their needs

    B. Identifying opportunities for improvement, proposing improvement initiatives, and measuring results

        1. Review of CQI tools

IV. CQI action steps

(In this section, explain the importance of staff involvement in CQI; emphasize the leading role employees will play as the program develops.)

    A. How the department will encourage ideas and input

    B. The department's CQI training and education program

    C. Forming CQI teams

V. Organizational and departmental CQI goals

(This section of your presentation should cover the CQI goals of your organization and your department. Encourage staff to voice their views.)

    A. Organizational and departmental CQI goals

    B. What CQI will mean for the HIM department

VI. Putting CQI to work in the HIM department

(Be specific about the implementation plans you have for the department. Solicit feedback from your staff and be available for questions and comments. See Chapter 5 for examples of how other HIM departments have used CQI.)

    A. Existing implementation plans

    B. Questions, comments, and ideas from the staff

Presentation overheads

The following pages contain sample presentation slides, which you can also use—along with the above outline—to develop your inservice presentation. Either photocopy them as is, or use them for inspiration as you're creating your own slides.

Continuous Quality Improvement (CQI)

From theory to practice...

...an inservice for the HIM department

CQI in context:

- Emerged from the management theories of W. Edwards Deming, which first gained popularity in Japan in the 1950s

- Took root in American business and industrial practices in the 1980s

- Continuous quality improvement becomes a requirement of the JCAHO in the late 1980s

- Significant support on our board for continuous quality improvement

- A key to success in the next century

- Let's get started!

The CQI mindset

Doing whatever it takes to ensure:

- **the best service**

- **the best outcome**

- **customer satisfaction**

- **employee satisfaction**

- **financial success**

The CQI mindset

Continuously examining processes and seeking opportunities for improvement that will:

- benefit customers

- improve our results

- make us more efficient

- maximize the quality of everything we do

CQI will allow us to reinvent our department continuously.

- **How do we want to operate?**

- **How do we want to relate to our customers?**

- **How do we want to relate to our colleagues?**

Key components of a CQI program:

- Analysis of our:

    - customers' needs and expectations

    - products

    - services

- Performance monitoring

- CQI teams

- Staff participation

Customer identification

- Who are our internal customers?

- Who are our external customers?

Customer needs and expectations

- Are we giving them what they want?

- Can we do better?

CQI tools

- **Improvement through data-driven change initiatives**

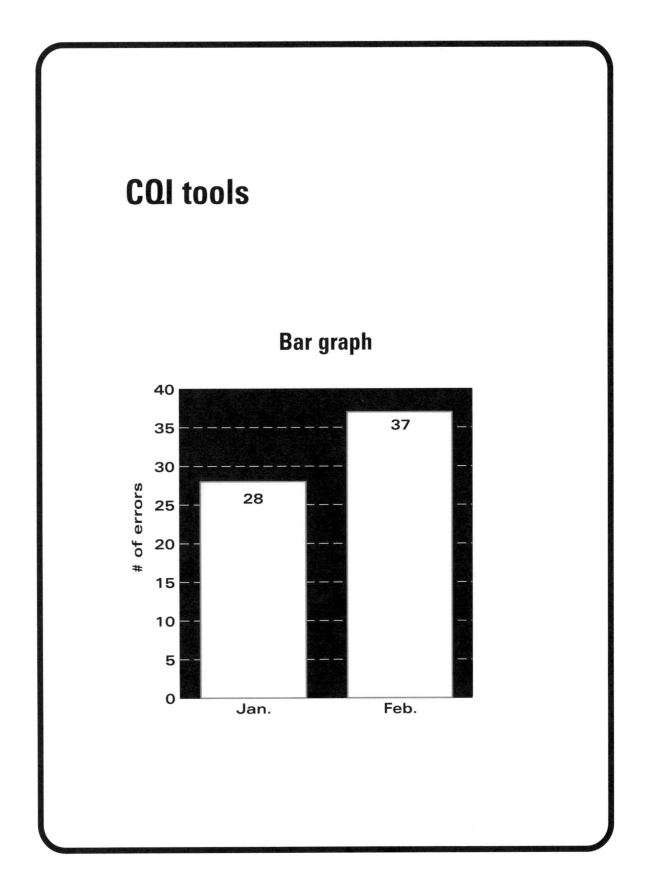

CQI tools

Bar graph

CQI tools

Cause-and-effect diagram

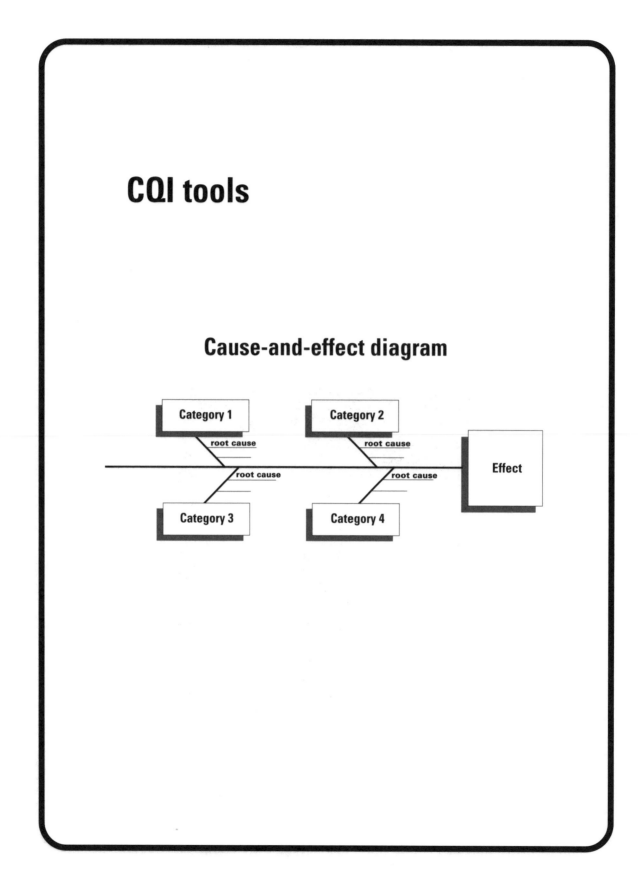

Continuous Quality Improvement for Health Information Management

CQI tools

Check sheets

Analysis errors						
Analysts \ Day	Mon	Tue	Wed	Thu	Fri	Weekly Total (Individuals)
Polly	✓✓✓		✓✓			5
Joe		✓				1
Sue	✓			✓✓		3
Daily Total (Dept.)	4	1	2	2	0	9

Major causes of incomplete records							
Causes	Frequency over six months						
Incomplete or missing:	Jan	Feb	March	April	May	June	Total
1. Histories & physicals	70	85	65	75	80	90	465
2. Attestations	140	150	135	145	160	170	900
3. Discharge summaries	125	130	140	135	130	130	790
4. Operative reports	60	80	95	90	120	100	545
5. Consultant reports	25	40	35	45	60	80	285
6. Signatures	150	165	170	155	170	200	1010
7. Other	80	50	70	35	40	70	345
Monthly Total	650	700	710	680	760	840	—

CQI tools

Decision matrix

Possible action steps for increasing transcription turnaround time

Rating system: 1=Unimportant   2=Important   3=Very Important

Alternatives	Criteria			Total	Rank
	Cost-Effective	Time to Implement	Acceptability		
Upgrade equipment	1	1	2	4	4
Use outside services	2	2	1	5	3
Develop incentives for transcriptionists	3	1	3	7	2
Hire a clerk to file, look up numbers, etc.	2	2	3	7	2
Hire two more transcriptionists	2	2	3	7	2
Stop typing non-clinical reports	3	3	3	9	1

CQI tools

Flow chart

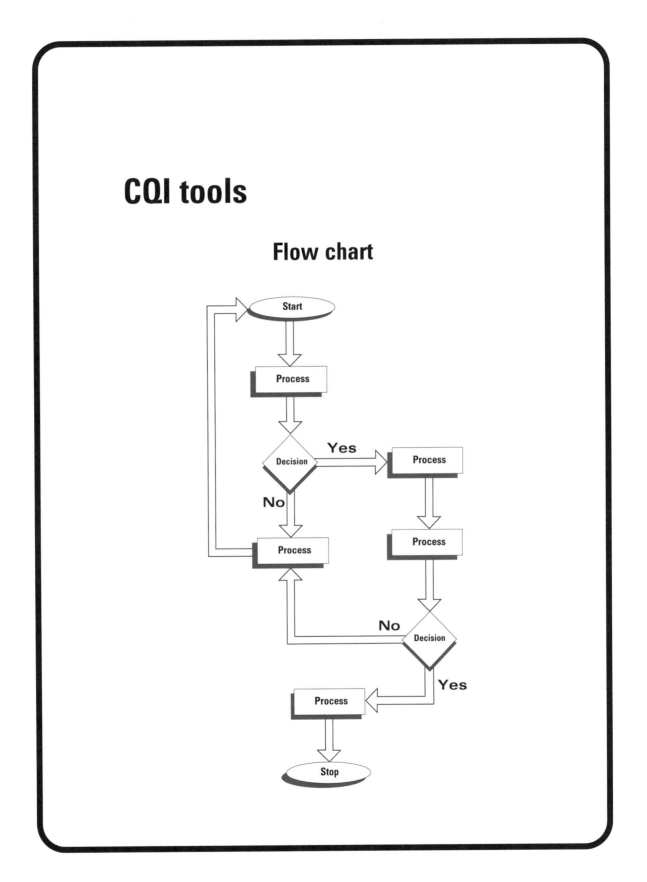

CQI tools

Histogram

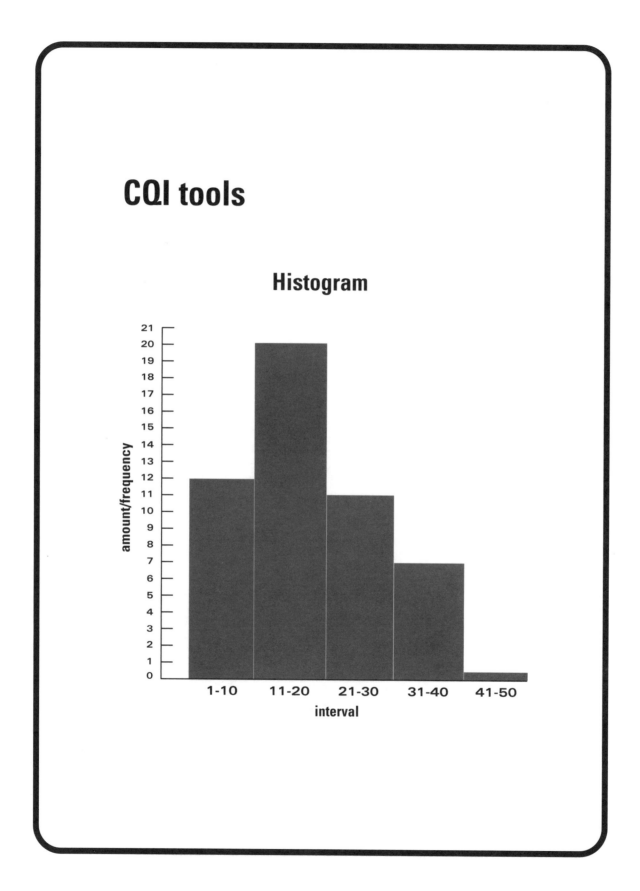

Continuous Quality Improvement for Health Information Management

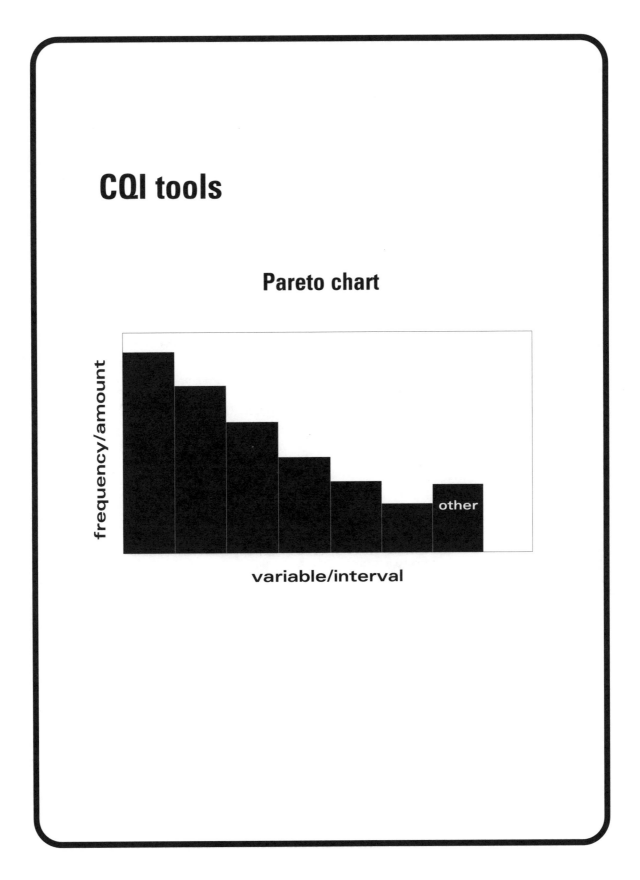

CQI tools

Pareto chart

CQI tools

PDCA method

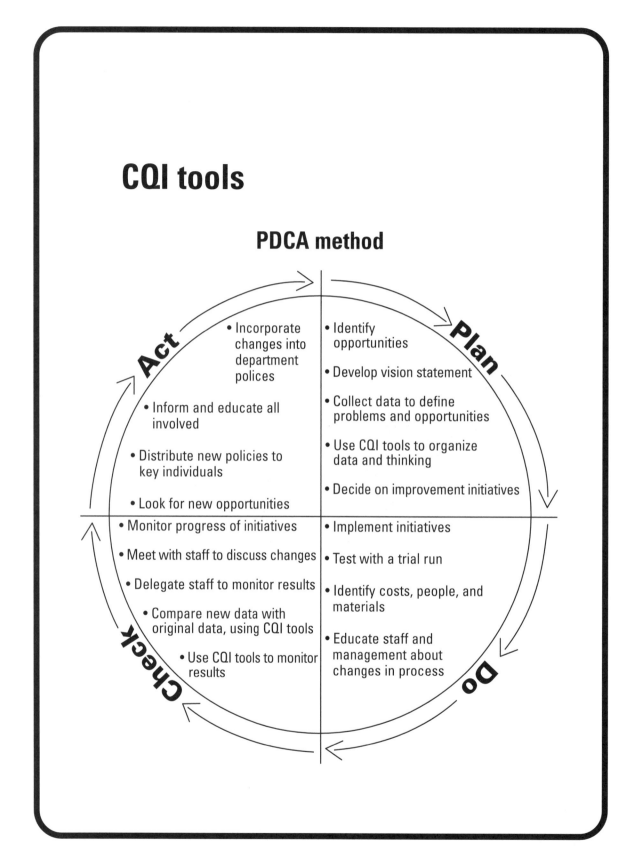

Act
- Incorporate changes into department polices
- Inform and educate all involved
- Distribute new policies to key individuals
- Look for new opportunities

Plan
- Identify opportunities
- Develop vision statement
- Collect data to define problems and opportunities
- Use CQI tools to organize data and thinking
- Decide on improvement initiatives

Check
- Monitor progress of initiatives
- Meet with staff to discuss changes
- Delegate staff to monitor results
- Compare new data with original data, using CQI tools
- Use CQI tools to monitor results

Do
- Implement initiatives
- Test with a trial run
- Identify costs, people, and materials
- Educate staff and management about changes in process

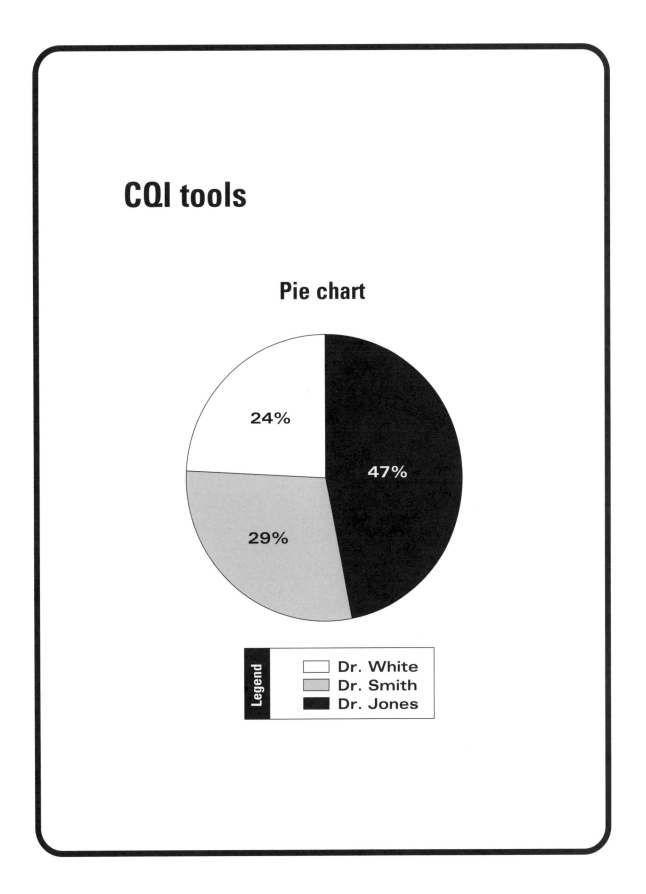

CQI tools

Pie chart

24%

47%

29%

Legend
☐ Dr. White
▨ Dr. Smith
■ Dr. Jones

CQI tools

Radar chart

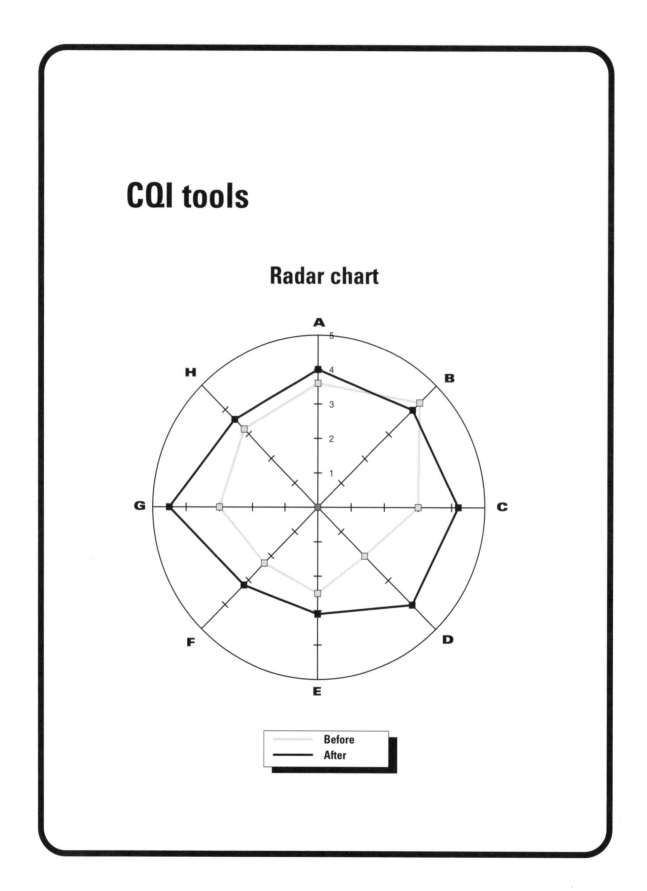

CQI tools

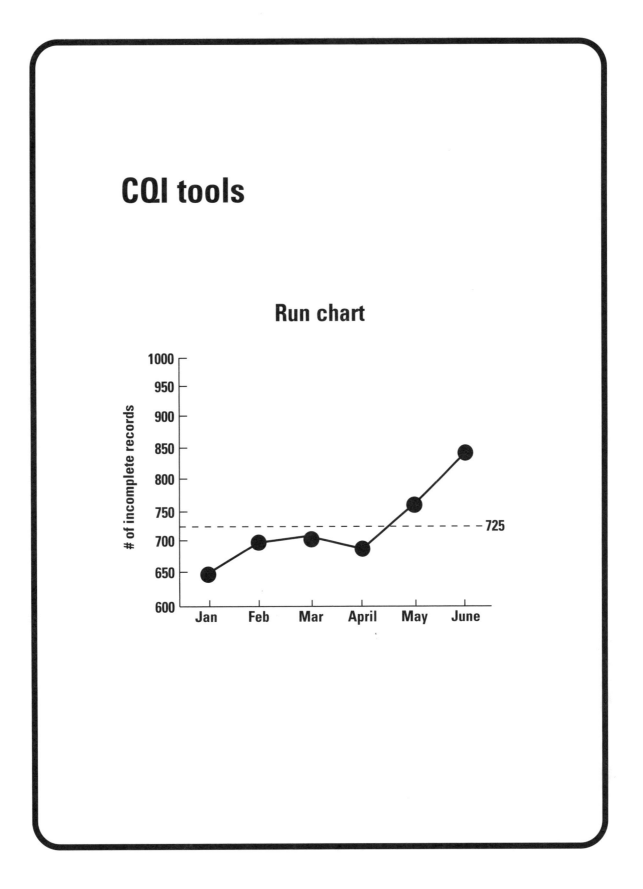

Run chart

CQI tools

Scatter diagram

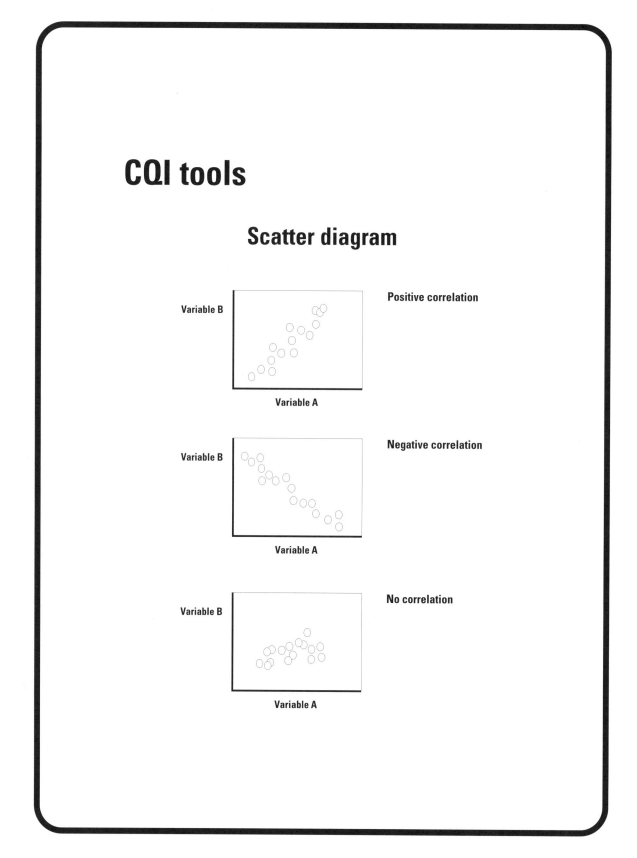

CQI action steps

- Educate and train
- Review existing documentation and policies
- Create department CQI implementation plan
- Update department policies and documentation
- Establish mechanisms for encouraging staff input
- Define departmental functions, services, and products
- Identify internal and external customers
- Identify customer needs and expectations
- Establish performance-monitoring mechanisms
- Establish CQI teams
- Identify and prioritize opportunities for improvement
- Track and share the results of improvement projects
- Modify criteria governing employee performance evaluations
- Continue improving

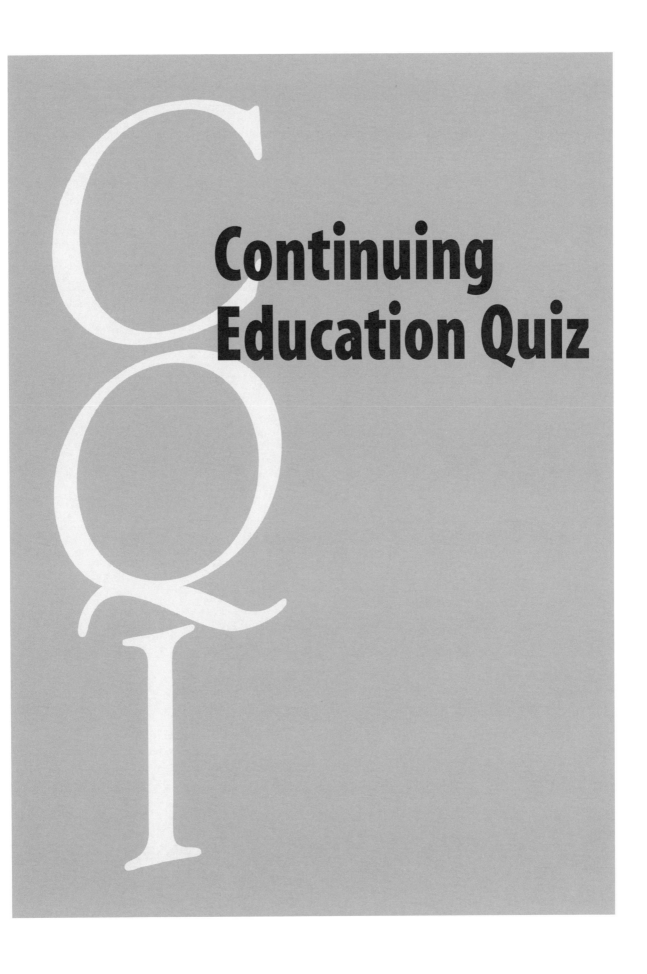

Continuing Education Quiz

Continuing Education Quiz

Directions

This is an open-book, multiple-choice quiz, with ten questions on each chapter of *Continuous Quality Improvement for Health Information Management*. Complete the answer sheet at the end of the quiz by clearly writing the letter that corresponds with your answer in the appropriate space. If more than one person in your organization is taking the quiz, photocopy as many blank answer sheets as you will need and have each person complete it separately. The information you will need to answer the questions can be found in the corresponding chapters of *Continuous Quality Improvement for Health Information Management*. You may refer back to these chapters as you take the quiz.

Return your answer sheet (please do not attach copies of the questions) to Opus Communications, along with a $35 payment for each person who completes the quiz. To qualify for the eight CE credit hours, you must get 75% of the answers correct— that's 53 out of 70 questions.

We'll send a certificate of completion to each person who passes the quiz, which may be used to document CE credits with the American Health Information Management Association (AHIMA).

This quiz has the approval of the AHIMA for eight (8) continuing education hours.

Chapter 1: Objectives of this Handbook

1. Health information management can affect _____.
   a. reimbursement
   b. accreditation
   c. patient care
   d. all of the above

2. The acronym "CQI" stands for _____.
   a. constant quality integration
   b. continuous quality improvement
   c. continuous quality intelligence
   d. constant quality ingenuity

3. Effective use of CQI means embracing a cycle of _____ that is designed to _____.
   a. reactive assessment/address visible problems
   b. reactive assessment/prevent problems
   c. continuous change/prevent problems
   d. quality monitoring/ensure problems

4. HIM departments that have truly embraced CQI _____.
   a. don't wait for problems to arise
   b. view it as a reactive process
   c. both of the above
   d. neither of the above

5. The handbook *Continuous Quality Improvement for Health Information Management* will help you become more knowledgeable about CQI by describing _____.
   a. shortcomings, tools, and concepts
   b. tools, methods, and means
   c. concepts, terms, and tools
   d. ideas, terms, and methods

6. Understanding the information in this handbook will help you _____.
   a. implement a CQI program in your department
   b. make CQI principles part of your department's culture
   c. both of the above
   d. neither of the above

7. CQI tools can help HIM departments _____.
   a. identify opportunities for improving processes
   b. develop improvement initiatives
   c. monitor improvement initiatives
   d. all of the above

8. The tools discussed in *Continuous Quality Improvement for Health Information Management* are an integral part of _____.
   a. new-home construction
   b. data-driven CQI
   c. Deming's 14 Points
   d. the Joiner Triangle

9. The quality concepts that gave rise to CQI were initially developed for _____.
   a. business and industry
   b. health information management
   c. the JCAHO
   d. all of the above

10. CQI can help you secure and protect _____ for your organization.
   a. Deming's 14 Points
   b. industry-wide respect
   c. money
   d. JCAHO accreditation

Chapter 2: CQI Basics

1. What is CQI?
    a. a data-driven process for improving performance
    b. a measure of intelligence
    c. quality assurance
    d. a means for determining an acceptable level of error

2. Of the following people, whose thinking helped shape CQI?
    a. Joseph M. Juran
    b. W. Edwards Deming
    c. Philip Crosby
    d. all of the above

3. Deming identified _____ points to help companies manage for maximum quality.
    a. 22
    b. 14
    c. 7
    d. 3

4. Juran's "Quality Trilogy" addresses which of the following processes?
    a. quality planning
    b. quality control
    c. quality improvement
    d. all of the above

5. According to Philip Crosby, quality should be _____.
    a. standards based
    b. legally mandated
    c. a national pastime
    d. none of the above

6. Deming and Crosby both emphasize that CQI should involve _____.
    a. everyone in an organization
    b. just management and senior management
    c. consultants
    d. patients

7. Joiner emphasizes training _____ to identify problems and opportunities, then training _____ to help propose and implement improvements.
    a. top management/patients
    b. employees/top management
    c. nurses/doctors
    d. top management/employees

8. According to Deming, what effect(s) do poorly handled merit ratings and annual reviews have?
    a. they create interest in and enthusiasm for quality improvement
    b. they prompt destructive competition, discourage teamwork, and damage employee morale
    c. they foster competition that leads to higher levels of performance
    d. they have no effect

9. The Joiner Triangle consists of which of the following?
    a. hypothesizing, testing, experimenting
    b. quality, peer review, reward system
    c. quality, scientific approach, all-one-team
    d. goal setting, infrastructure, resources

10. According to Joiner, _____ is the key to CQI.
    a. teamwork
    b. production
    c. budgeting
    d. change

Chapter 3: Applying CQI to HIM

1. Deming's first point requires that HIM departments _____.
   a. demonstrate effective use of CQI
   b. eliminate chart delinquencies
   c. know their customers
   d. ignore their customers

2. Deming's third point implies that quality programs should be _____.
   a. evaluated quarterly
   b. proactive not reactive
   c. dependent on mass inspection
   d. none of the above

3. According to Deming's eleventh point, quotas are probably a poor way to

   _____.
   a. increase quality and accuracy
   b. improve employee performance
   c. both of the above
   d. neither of the above

4. Why is it important to establish a complaint tracking system?
   a. it will help employees overcome their fear of raising negative issues publicly
   b. it will help your department spot opportunities for improvement
   c. both of the above
   d. neither of the above

5. Employee performance standards should be _____.
   a. draconian
   b. qualitative not quantitative
   c. flexible and optional
   d. changed constantly

6. An HIM department's customer list should include _____.
   a. everyone who depends upon the department's information and services
   b. external customers
   c. internal customers
   d. all of the above

7. Which of the following devices can help you capture suggestions?
   a. a suggestion box
   b. an idea board
   c. both of the above
   d. neither of the above

8. Recognizing employee contributions to CQI efforts is important because

   _____.
   a. it's the polite thing to do
   b. it demonstrates management support for CQI without taking control of the process away from employees
   c. JCAHO standards require such recognition
   d. none of the above

9. The JCAHO requires facilities to _____ data on patient care, treatment outcomes, and other key functions.
   a. measure and assess
   b. manipulate
   c. ignore
   d. share with other facilities

10. An organization's main goal in implementing CQI should be to _____.
    a. satisfy JCAHO accreditation requirements
    b. improve patient care
    c. hold more meetings
    d. none of the above

Chapter 4: CQI Tools

1. If you wish to generate as many ideas as possible on a particular subject, which CQI tool should you use?
    a. scatter diagram
    b. flow chart
    c. brainstorming
    d. customer satisfaction survey

2. How does Nominal Group Technique differ from brainstorming?
    a. NGT uses an objective rating system to prioritize ideas
    b. NGT elicits responses from a group of people
    c. NGT uses a chalkboard or flip chart to keep track of responses
    d. NGT can be done by mail

3. A flow chart identifies _____.
    a. steps in a decision
    b. steps in a process
    c. customer needs
    d. customer satisfaction

4. How does a survey differ from an interview?
    a. responses may be written
    b. there is less opportunity for variation
    c. both of the above
    d. neither of the above

5. A histogram displays _____.
    a. patterns of occurrence over time
    b. categories of data from largest to smallest
    c. patient allergies
    d. priorities

6. Check sheets do NOT identify _____.

    a. causes

    b. how often an event occurs

    c. patient name

    d. all of the above

7. Which of the following could be plotted with data from a check sheet?

    a. a histogram

    b. a pareto chart

    c. a run chart

    d. all of the above

8. A CQI team could use _____ to prioritize its options.

    a. a flow chart

    b. the PDCA method

    c. a decision matrix

    d. a customer satisfaction survey

9. In the final phase of the PDCA method, how should a department institutionalize effective changes?

    a. by revising relevant policies

    b. by firing employees who resist the changes

    c. by notifying the JCAHO

    d. by alerting patients and news media

10. A cause and effect diagram is sometimes called _____.

    a. a fishbone diagram

    b. an Ishikawa diagram

    c. both of the above

    d. neither of the above

Chapter 5: Case Studies

1. What CQI tool helped Fairview Clinics identify that reliance on handwritten completion was a potential reason for inaccurate or incomplete charge tickets?
   a. brainstorming
   b. surveys
   c. flow charts
   d. the PDCA method

2. What did Fairview hope would result from its standardization efforts?
   a. less confusion
   b. less rework
   c. increased reimbursement
   d. all of the above

3. What helps Morton Plant Mease Health Care monitor indicators continuously?
   a. bar coding and computers
   b. cellular telephones
   c. closed circuit television
   d. none of the above

4. What tool allowed Morton Plant Mease to improve the accuracy of attending-physician designations on patient charts?
   a. survey
   b. check sheet
   c. flow chart
   d. histogram

5. What tool allowed the CQI team at Morton Plant Mease to track trends in chart delinquencies and physician suspensions over several months?
   a. flow charts
   b. radar charts
   c. pareto charts
   d. run charts

6. How does Roper's FOCUS PDCA method differ from the traditional PDCA method?
   a. it is more focused and intense
   b. it separates preliminary analysis used to identify possible improvement initiatives from activities involved in implementing those initiatives
   c. it doesn't differ
   d. none of the above

7. Why did the CQI team at Roper employ a cause-and-effect diagram?
   a. it helped categorize their list of possible actions and made it more manageable
   b. it helped them brainstorm potential improvement initiatives
   c. to design its FOCUS PDCA method
   d. all of the above

8. In the Roper case study, what does the bar graph in Figure 7 show?
   a. the time that the CQI team spent on analysis
   b. that on-time returns jumped from 11 percent in April 1996 to 90 percent by April 1997
   c. that physicians alone were to blame for late signatures on plans of care
   d. none of the above

9. Why was the HIM director at Harris Methodist Fort Worth interested in reducing the number of chart requests that came from databases and registries?
   a. because the databases and registries are not important
   b. so his staff could take more vacation time
   c. because the requests reduced the time spent fulfilling treatment-related requests, completing charts, and supporting billing
   d. none of the above

10. Why did Harris Methodist weight its decision matrix criteria (Figure 3b)?
    a. so the most important criteria would have more effect on the overall priority rating
    b. so the ideas of senior employees would be implemented first
    c. to weed out bad ideas from a list of improvement initiatives
    d. all of the above

Chapter 6: CQI Planner

1. Managers who wish to establish a CQI program for their HIM department should first educate _____.
   a. their staff
   b. themselves
   c. their CEO
   d. W. Edwards Deming

2. To design an effective CQI program, managers must be willing to _____.
   a. resign if their plans are rejected
   b. fire employees who resist their plans
   c. grant significant autonomy to staff
   d. all of the above

3. Which of the following is/are among the documents that should be assembled before an HIM department attempts to draft a CQI plan?
   a. a patient bill of rights
   b. patient care plan
   c. information management plan
   d. all organizational vision statements relevant to CQI, quality, performance improvement, and/or customer service

4. Which of the following might help you educate staff about CQI tools, techniques, and principles?
   a. a suggestion box and idea board
   b. inservice sessions and a CQI reading club
   c. all of the above
   d. none of the above

5. Which of the following things should you identify to assist development of a CQI plan?
   a. your department's functions, services, and products
   b. your department's internal and external customers
   c. your customers' needs and expectations
   d. all of the above

6. _____ are/is a key component of CQI.
   a. lunch meetings
   b. ongoing performance monitoring
   c. poor performance
   d. none of the above

7. If your initial analysis identifies more opportunities for improvement than your department is prepared to address, which of the following tools might help you set priorities?
   a. cause-and-effect diagrams, decision matrices, and pareto charts
   b. brainstorming and scatter diagrams
   c. radar charts, run charts, and histograms
   d. flow charts

8. Why might it be good to include people from outside the HIM department on your CQI team?
   a. so your employees won't have to interrupt their work day
   b. because they know more about HIM processes
   c. because they can offer fresh perspectives and insights
   d. so you can network

9. Departments that have embraced CQI often modify performance-evaluation measures for employees, making them _____.
   a. optional
   b. qualitative, not quantitative
   c. nonexistent
   d. quantitative, not qualitative

10. Once your CQI program is up and running, encourage managers and staff to look for improvement opportunities _____.
    a. periodically
    b. when instructed to do so
    c. during an initial brainstorming session
    d. constantly

Chapter 7: CQI Inservice Kit

1. When conducting an inservice, keep in mind that people absorb information _____, but _____ generally enhance a presentation.
    a. in different ways/slides, handouts, and reading material
    b. in the same way/printed handouts
    c. quickly/a fast overview of CQI philosophy and methods
    d. slowly/a gradual introduction to CQI philosophy and methods

2. To give a quick overview of CQI, plan an inservice _____.
    a. that lasts about an hour and covers the basics
    b. that leaves time for identifying customers
    c. that lasts about half an hour and includes slides
    d. that includes development of a CQI team and identification of improvement initiatives

3. Which of the following is NOT a "trick of the trade" for public speaking?
    a. know your subject
    b. use real-life examples
    c. be enthusiastic
    d. read from a script

4. Which "trick of the trade" helps you become comfortable with your material and allows you to focus, during your presentation, on delivering that material engagingly?
    a. don't rely on notes
    b. move around and encourage audience participation
    c. practice, practice, practice
    d. don't rush

5. If you use notes during your presentation, be sure they _____.
    a. are large and easy to read—since you'll be relying heavily on them
    b. cover major points, but don't script your talk completely
    c. are grammatically correct
    d. none of the above

6. Why are real-life examples and anecdotes effective in a presentation?
    a. they are not effective
    b. they put the topic in a meaningful context
    c. they're funny
    d. none of the above

7. Moving around during a presentation is a good way to _____.
    a. settle your nerves
    b. boost your energy and enthusiasm
    c. keep your audience engaged
    d. all of the above

8. How can visual aids help a presentation?
    a. they can illustrate complex material
    b. they can help hold the audience's attention
    c. they can help the presenter stay focused and on track
    d. all of the above

9. Pausing briefly during a presentation _____.
    a. helps drive your key points home
    b. makes your audience nervous
    c. makes you look stupid
    d. gives you a chance to take a sip of water

10. A few minutes before your presentation begins, you should _____.
    a. rewrite it completely
    b. breathe and relax
    c. rehearse one last time
    d. check the grammar in your notes

Answer Sheet

We suggest that you photocopy this page and use the copy for your responses. Please write the letter corresponding to your answer in the appropriate space below.

Chapter One	Chapter Two	Chapter Three	Chapter Four	Chapter Five	Chapter Six	Chapter Seven
1._____	1._____	1._____	1._____	1._____	1._____	1._____
2._____	2._____	2._____	2._____	2._____	2._____	2._____
3._____	3._____	3._____	3._____	3._____	3._____	3._____
4._____	4._____	4._____	4._____	4._____	4._____	4._____
5._____	5._____	5._____	5._____	5._____	5._____	5._____
6._____	6._____	6._____	6._____	6._____	6._____	6._____
7._____	7._____	7._____	7._____	7._____	7._____	7._____
8._____	8._____	8._____	8._____	8._____	8._____	8._____
9._____	9._____	9._____	9._____	9._____	9._____	9._____
10._____	10._____	10._____	10._____	10._____	10._____	10._____

Check one: ❑ ART   ❑ RRA   ❑ Other (please specify) _____

Name _____

Address _____

City _____ State _____ Zip _____

Telephone _____

AHIMA (AMRA) ID # _____

Please enclose a check for $35 payable to Opus Communications for each answer sheet being submitted. Mail to:

Opus Communications, P.O. Box 1168, Marblehead, MA 01945

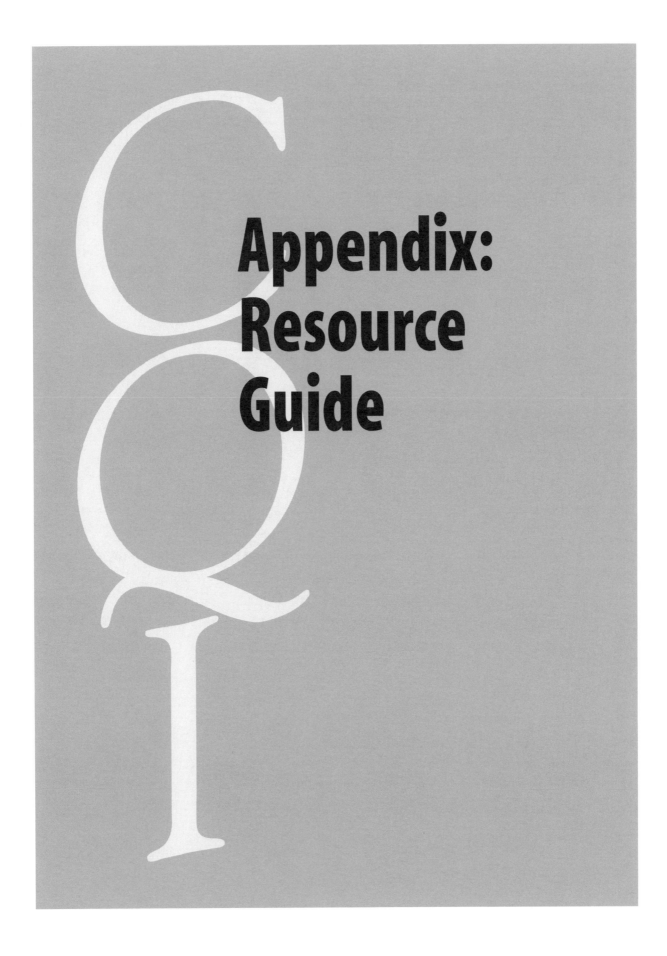

Appendix: Resource Guide

Appendix: Resource Guide

Organizations

American Society for Quality Control
611 East Wisconsin Avenue
Milwaukee, WI 53202
Telephone: 414/272-8575
Fax: 414/272-1734
- publishes the book *Quality Improvement*
- publishes the newsletter *Quality Progress*

Association for Quality and Participation
801B West Eighth Street, Suite 501
Cincinnati, OH 45203
Telephone: 513/381-1959
Fax: 513/381-0070
- publishes *The Journal for Quality and Participation*
- publishes *News for Change*

Care Education Group
2 Salt Lake Creek
Hinsdale, IL 60521
Telephone: 630/323-1900
Fax: 630/323-2123
- publishes material on quality assurance and quality improvement
- provides consulting services

Goal/QPC
13 Branch Street
Methuen, MA 01844
Telephone: 978/685-3900
Fax: 978/685-6151
- CQI videos, books, and seminars

Institute for Healthcare Improvement

135 Francis Street

Boston, MA 02215

Telephone: 617/424-4800

Fax: 617/754-4848

- CQI seminars

Juran Institute, Inc.

11 River Road

Wilton, CT 06897

Telephone: 203/834-1700

Fax: 203/834-9891

- CQI books, seminars, and consulting services

Productivity

101 Merritt #7

Norwalk, CT 06851

Telephone: 800/966-5423

Fax: 203/846-6883

- publishes the newsletter TEI: *Total Employee Involvement*

Periodicals

The Joint Commission Journal on Quality Improvement

Joint Commission on Accreditation of Healthcare Organizations

One Renaissance Boulevard

Oakbrook Terrace, IL 60181

Telephone: 630/792-5000

Fax: 630/792-5005

Journal for Healthcare Quality

National Association for Healthcare Quality

4700 West Lake Avenue

Glenview, IL 60025-1485

Telephone: 800/966-9392

Fax: 847/375-4777

Perspectives: The Official Joint Commission Newsletter
Joint Commission on Accreditation of Healthcare Organizations
One Renaissance Boulevard
Oakbrook Terrace, IL 60181
Telephone: 630/792-5000
Fax: 630/792-5005

QI-TQM
American Health Consultants
P.O. Box 740056
Atlanta, GA 30374-0056
Telephone: 404/262-7436
Fax: 404/262-7837

Quality Digest
QCI International
17055 Quail Ridge Road
Cottonwood, CA 96022
Telephone: 530/347-1334
Fax: 530/347-6987

Quality Management in Health Care
Aspen Publishers, Inc.
7201 McKinney Circle
Frederick, MD 21701
Telephone: 800/234-1660
Fax: 800/901-9075

The Quality Observer
Quality Observer Corporation
P.O. Box 1111
Fairfax, VA 22030
Telephone: 703/691-9496
Fax: 703/691-9399

Topics in Health Information Management: Quality and Performance Improvement
Volume 18, Number 3, February 1998
Aspen Publishers, Inc.
7201 McKinney Circle
Frederick, MD 21701
Telephone: 800/234-1660
Fax: 800/901-9075

Total Quality Newsletter
Lakewood Publications
50 South Ninth Street
Minneapolis, MN 55402
Telephone: 800/328-4329
Fax: 612/333-6526

Books

Albrecht, Karl. *At America's Service: How Your Company Can Join the Customer Service Revolution*. New York: Warner Books, 1995.

——. *The Only Thing That Matters*. New York: Harper Business, 1993.

Asaka, T. and K. Ozeki, eds. *Handbook of Quality Tools*. Cambridge: Productivity Press, 1990.

Belasco, J. A. *Teaching the Elephant to Dance: The Manager's Guide to Empowering Change*. New York: Crown Publishers, Inc., 1990.

Bennis, W. *On Becoming a Leader*. New York: Addison-Wesley, 1989.

Berry, Leonard L. and A. Parasuraman. *Marketing Services: Competing Through Quality*. New York: The Free Press, 1991.

Berry, T. H. *Managing the Total Quality Transformation*. New York: McGraw-Hill, 1991.

Berwick, D. M., et al. *Curing Health Care: New Strategies for Quality Improvement*. San Francisco: Jossey-Bass, 1990.

Brassard, Michael. *The Memory Jogger Plus*. Madison, WI: Joiner Associates, 1989.

Camp, Robert C. *Benchmarking: The Search for Industry Best Practices That Lead to Superior Performance*. Milwaukee: ASQC Quality Press, 1989.

Carey, Raymond G. and Robert C. Lloyd. *Measuring Quality Improvement in Healthcare: A Guide to Statistical Process Control Applications*. New York: Quality Resources, 1995.

Carr, Maureen P. and Francis W. Jackson. *The Crosswalk: Joint Commission Standards and Baldridge Criteria*. Oakbrook, IL: Joint Commission on Accreditation of Healthcare Organizations, 1997.

Cesarone, Diane. *Assess for Success: Achieving Excellence with Joint Commission Standards and Baldridge Criteria*. Oakbrook, IL: Joint Commission on Accreditation of Healthcare Organizations, 1997.

Crosby, Philip. *Quality Is Free: The Art of Making Quality Certain*. New York: New American Library, 1979.

————. *Quality Without Tears*. New York: McGraw-Hill, 1984.

————. *The Eternally Successful Organization: The Art of Corporate Wellness*. New York: McGraw-Hill, 1988.

Davidow, William H. and Bro Uttal. *Total Customer Service, the Ultimate Weapon: A Six-Point Plan for Giving Your Business the Competitive Edge in the 1990s*. New York: Harper & Row, 1989.

Deming, W. E. *Out of the Crisis*. Cambridge: Massachusetts Institute of Technology, Center for Advanced Engineering Study, 1986.

Feigenbaum, Armand V. *Total Quality Control*, 3rd ed. New York: McGraw-Hill, 1983.

Gabor, A. *The Man Who Discovered Quality*. New York: Times Books/Random House, 1990.

Gaucher, E. and R. Coffey. *Transforming Healthcare Organizations*. San Francisco: Jossey-Bass, 1990.

Garvin, David A. *Managing Quality: The Strategic and Competitive Edge*. New York: The Free Press, 1988.

Geehr, E. C. and J. Pine, eds. *Increasing Physician Involvement in Quality Improvement Programs*. Tampa: The American College of Physician Executives, 1992.

Gitlow, H. S. *Planning for Quality, Productivity, and Competitive Position*. Chicago: Irwin Professional Publishing, 1990.

——— , et al. *Tools and Methods for the Improvement of Quality*. Homewood: Dow Jones-Irwin Publishers, 1989.

GOAL/QPC. *The Memory Jogger: A Pocket Guide of Tools for Continuous Improvement and Effective Planning*. Methuen, MA: GOAL/QPC, 1994.

GOAL/QPC. *The Team Memory Jogger*. Methuen, MA: GOAL/QPC, 1995

Goldratt, E. M. and J. Cox. *The Goal: A Process of Ongoing Improvement*. Croton-on-Hudson, NY: North River Press, 1994.

Guaspari, John. *Theory Why*. New York: American Management Association, 1986.

Harrison, H. J. *Business Process Improvement: The Breakthrough Strategy for Total Quality, Productivity and Competitiveness*. New York: McGraw-Hill, 1991.

Hartzler, Meg and Jane E. Henry, PhD. *Team Fitness: A How-To Manual for Building a Winning Work Team*. Milwaukee: ASQC Press, 1994.

Hospital Corporation of America. *Hospitalwide Quality Technology Network*. Nashville: HCA, 1991.

Imai, Masaki. *Kaizen: The Key to Japan's Competitive Success*. New York: Random House, 1986.

Ishikawa, Kaoru. *Guide to Quality Control*. Tokyo: Asian Productivity Organization, 1982.

JCAHO. *Comprehensive Accreditation Manual for Hospitals*. Oakbrook Terrace, IL: Joint Commission on Accreditation of Healthcare Organizations, 1997.

JCAHO. *Exploring Quality Improvement Principles: A Hospital Leader's Guide*. Oakbrook Terrace, IL: Joint Commission on Accreditation of Healthcare Organizations, 1992.

JCAHO. *Framework for Improving Performance: From Principles to Practice*. Oakbrook Terrace, IL: Joint Commission on Accreditation of Healthcare Organizations, 1994.

JCAHO. *Implementing Quality Improvement: A Hospital Leader's Guide*. Oakbrook Terrace, IL: Joint Commission on Accreditation of Healthcare Organizations, 1993.

JCAHO. *Introduction to Quality Improvement in Health Care*. Oakbrook Terrace, IL: Joint Commission on Accreditation of Healthcare Organizations, 1991.

JCAHO. *A Pocket Guide to Quality Improvement Tools*. Oakbrook Terrace, IL: Joint Commission on Accreditation of Healthcare Organizations, 1992.

JCAHO. *Primer on Indicator Development and Application: Measuring Quality in Health Care*. Oakbrook Terrace, IL: Joint Commission on Accreditation of Healthcare Organizations, 1990.

JCAHO. *Process Improvement Models: Case Studies in Health Care*. Oakbrook Terrace, IL: Joint Commission on Accreditation of Healthcare Organizations, 1993.

JCAHO. *Striving Toward Improvement: Six Hospitals in Search of Quality*. Oakbrook Terrace, IL: Joint Commission on Accreditation of Healthcare Organizations, 1992.

JCAHO. *The Transition from QA to CQI: An Introduction to Quality Improvement in Health Care*. Oakbrook Terrace, IL: Joint Commission on Accreditation of Healthcare Organizations, 1991.

JCAHO. *Transitions: From QA to CQI—Using CQI Approaches to Monitor, Evaluate, and Improve Quality*. Oakbrook Terrace, IL: Joint Commission on Accreditation of Healthcare Organizations, 1991.

JCAHO. *Using Quality Improvement Tools in a Health Care Setting.* Oakbrook Terrace, IL: Joint Commission on Accreditation of Healthcare Organizations, 1992.

James, B. C. *Quality Management for Health Care Delivery.* Chicago: Hospital Research and Educational Trust, 1988.

——. *Total Quality Leadership vs. Management by Results.* Madison, WI: Joiner Associates, 1985.

Juran, J. M. *Juran on Leadership for Quality: An Executive Handbook.* New York: The Free Press, 1989.

——. *Juran on Planning for Quality.* New York: The Free Press, 1988.

—— and F. M. Gryna. *Juran's Quality Control Handbook,* 4th ed. New York: McGraw-Hill, 1988.

Kieffer, George David. *The Strategy of Meetings.* New York: Warner, 1988.

King, B. *Hoshin Planning: The Developmental Approach.* Methuen, MA: GOAL/QPC, 1989.

Kotter, John P. *The Leadership Factor.* New York: The Free Press, 1988.

Kouzes, James M. and Barry Z. Pozner. *The Leadership Challenge.* San Francisco: Jossey-Bass, 1987.

Kriegel, Robert J. and Louis Patler. *If It Ain't Broke, Break It.* New York: Warner, 1991.

—— and David Brandt. *Sacred Cows Make the Best Burgers: Developing Change-Ready People and Organizations.* New York: Warner Books, 1997.

Leebov, Wendy. *The Quality Quest.* Chicago: American Hospital Publishing, 1991.

——. *Service Excellence: The Customer Relations Strategy for Health Care.* Chicago: American Hospital Publishing, 1988.

—— and Clara Jean Ersoz. *The Health Care Manager's Guide to Continuous Quality Improvement*. Chicago: American Hospital Publishing, 1991.

—— and G. Scott. *Health Care Managers in Transition: Shifting Roles and Changing Organizations*. San Francisco: Jossey-Bass, 1990.

Lefevre, Henry L. *Quality Service Pays: Six Keys to Success!* Milwaukee: ASQC Quality Press, 1989.

Lele, Milind M. and Jagdish N. Sheth. *The Customer Is Key*. New York: John Wiley & Sons, 1987.

Lieberman, Ernest D. *Unfit to Manage*. New York: McGraw-Hill, 1988.

Melum, Mara Minerva and Marie Kuchuris Sinioris. *Total Quality Management: The Health Care Pioneers*. Chicago: American Hospital Publishing, 1992.

Moran, John W., Casey Collett, and Claudette Cote. *Daily Management: A System for Individual and Organizational Optimization*. Methuen, MA: GOAL/QPC, 1991.

——, Richard P. Talbot, and Russell M. Benson. *A Guide to Graphical Problem-Solving Processes*. Milwaukee: ASQC Quality Press, 1990.

Nadler, G., and S. Hibino. *Breakthrough Thinking*. Rocklin, CA: Prima Publishing, 1998.

Naisbitt, John. *Megatrends*. New York: Warner Books, 1988.

Noble, Sara P. *301 Great Management Ideas from America's Most Innovative Small Companies*. Boston: Goldhersh Group, 1991.

Omachonu, Vincent K. *Total Quality and Productivity Management in Health Care Organizations*. Milwaukee: Institute of Industrial Engineers and the ASQC Quality Press, 1991.

Opus Communications. *The JCAHO Survey Coordinator's Handbook*. Marblehead, MA: Opus Communications, 1997.

Peters, Thomas. *Thriving on Chaos*. New York: Harper & Row, 1987.

—— and Robert H. Waterman. *In Search of Excellence*. New York: Harper & Row, 1982.

Psarouthakis, J. *Better Makes Us Best*. Cambridge: Productivity Press, 1989.

Rosander, A. C. *The Quest for Quality in Services*. Milwaukee: ASQC Quality Press, 1989.

————. *Deming's 14 Points Applied to Services*. Milwaukee: ASQC Press, 1991.

Scholtes, P. R., et al. *The TEAM Handbook*. Madison, WI: Joiner Associates, 1988.

Shewhart, Walter. *Economic Control of Quality of Manufactured Product*. New York: Van Nostrand, 1931.

Shigeru, M. *Management for Quality Improvement*. Cambridge: Productivity Press, 1989.

Spath, Patrice, ed. *Innovations in Health Care Quality Measurement*. Chicago: American Hospital Publishing, 1989.

Steiber, S. and W. Krowinski. *Measuring and Managing Patient Satisfaction*. Chicago: American Hospital Publishing, 1990. '

Walton, Mary. *Deming Management at Work*. New York: Putnam, 1990.

——. *The Deming Management Method*. New York: Putnam, 1986.

Audio-Visual Resources

Charthouse Learning Corporation
221 River Ridge Circle
Burnsville, MN 55337
Telephone: 800/328-3789
Fax: 612/890-0505
  • *The Business of Paradigms* (video)
  • *The Power of Vision* (video)

Web Sites

American Society for Quality—Health Care Division
http://www.asqc.org

American Customer Satisfaction Index
http://acsi.asqc.org

National Quality Program
home of the Malcolm Baldrige National Quality Award
http://www.quality.nist.gov

Site for *The Quarterly Journal of Cost and Quality*
http://www.cost-quality.com

The National Committee for Quality Assurance
http://www.ncqa.org

The Joint Commission on Accreditation of Healthcare Organizations
http://www.jcaho.org

The Agency for Health Care Policy Research
http://www.ahcpr.gov

The American Productivity & Quality Center
http://www.apqc.org

U.S. Department of Health and Human Services
http://www.os.dhhs.gov

National Institutes of Health
http://www.nih.gov

The National Network of Libraries of Medicine
http://www.nnlm.nlm.nih.gov/nnlmlist.html

National Center for Health Statistics
http://www.cdc.gov/nchswww

Consumer Coalition for Quality Health Care
http://www.consumers.org

Related Products from Opus Communications, The Greeley Company, and The Greeley Education Company

Newsletters

Medical Records Briefing

Medical Records Briefing is a respected monthly newsletter that covers the latest developments, important trends, and innovative ideas in the field of health information management. Each issue is full of crucial information, such as the latest Medicare changes; practical advice on tough legal, financial, and human-resources issues; and real-life HIM success stories. Subscribers have an opportunity to earn 12 continuing-education credits through the newsletter's biannual CE quizzes.

Free subscriber benefits include:
- "MRB Talk"—an Internet discussion group where readers network with peers; and
- Fax Express—When news can't wait for the next monthly issue, subscribers automatically receive special faxed alerts.

Health Information Management Across the Continuum

Whether they work in home care, ambulatory care, physicians' offices, long-term care, subacute care, rehabilitation, or assisted living, subscribers to Health Information Management Across the Continuum receive news and advice that meets their HIM needs. Monthly newsletter issues and monthly binder-section supplements also look at ways of integrating HIM functions across healthcare settings.

Free subscriber benefits include:
- "MRB Talk"—an Internet discussion group where readers network with peers; and
- Fax Express—When news can't wait, subscribers automatically receive special faxed alerts.

Briefings on Coding Compliance Strategies

Briefings on Coding Compliance Strategies provides subscribers with information and advice on meeting requirements for coding, documentation, and billing. This monthly publication offers ideas and insights—from peers, consultants, and other professionals—on complying with the rules of Medicare and private insurers.

Free subscriber benefits include:
- "CCO Talk"—an Internet discussion group where readers network with their peers; and
- Fax Express—When news can't wait for the next monthly issue, subscribers automatically receive special faxed alerts.

Books

Mastering Records Completion: Successful Strategies from Medical Records Briefing

This exciting book is a compilation of the best articles on records-completion strategies from ten years of *Medical Records Briefing*. *Mastering Records Completion* explores the "big-picture" skills that HIM professionals need to master this critical function and to fulfill JCAHO records-completion requirements. Its five chapters offer articles, interviews, and cutting-edge advice from industry experts, and each chapter includes the best tips and strategies that *Medical Records Briefing* has to offer.

Information Management: The Compliance Guide to the JCAHO Standards, Second Edition

This hands-on compliance guide offers advice and information you'll need to weather a JCAHO survey. It provides straightforward analysis of the JCAHO's IM standards, and it includes detailed, practical advice on how to develop an information-management plan, how to improve HIM functions, and how to prepare your department for a JCAHO survey. *Information Management* also includes a continuing-education quiz that allows you to earn 6 CE credits at a fraction of the cost you would normally pay.

12 Weeks to a Successful Data Dictionary

This book takes a straightforward look at a difficult, technical subject: building a data dictionary. It outlines a 12-week approach that you can commit to and complete successfully. You'll learn how to:
- consolidate your organization's information resources to improve the consistency and accuracy with which you analyze, display, and report data;
- select an interdepartmental project team to create your data dictionary;
- comply with the JCAHO's IM.3 standard;
- understand and create data fields; and
- develop and implement a database infrastructure that can survive growth, mergers, and acquisitions—one that your organization can bank on for the future.

NetPractice™: A Beginner's Guide to Healthcare Networking on the Internet

by Mary Frances Miller, MS, RRA

This instructional guide is designed to give everyone in your organization—from medical-staff professionals and information managers to physicians and nurses—a no-nonsense introduction to browsing the Internet. User-friendly, *NetPractice* ™ will not overwhelm you with Internet services, jargon, and protocols. It explores common and practical uses of the Internet—like on-line global communications through e-mail, mailing lists, newsgroups, and the World Wide Web. It also includes free starter kits from CompuServe and America Online that offer 10 free hours of on-line service.

Videos

It's Everybody's Job—A Team-Based Approach to Medical Records Completion

Accurate and timely records completion is critical to providing quality patient care, achieving compliance with accreditation and regulatory standards, and expediting patient billing. That's why *It's Everybody's Job—A Team-Based Approach to Medical Records Completion* is the ideal starting point if you want to create or improve a records-completion program. This dynamic, 14-minute training video is the perfect springboard for starting, rekindling, or perpetuating effective dialog with your medical staff. The video includes ideas and insights from HIM directors, administrators, CEOs, and physicians. Learn their strategies for expediting authentication and completion of discharge documents, for streamlining processes and systems, and for developing effective records-completion policies. You'll also learn how they encourage initiative from and motivate their medical staffs.

Keep it to Yourself! Protecting Patient Confidentiality

As medical records and other sources of patient information are computerized, the task of maintaining patient confidentiality is becoming more challenging than ever. That's why The Greeley Education Company and Harvard Pilgrim Health Care collaborated on *Keep it to Yourself! Protecting Patient Confidentiality*, a 14-minute training video that is designed to attune your staff to the importance of safeguarding confidential patient information. You'll learn about common mistakes and slips that can breach confidentiality, and you'll get advice on how to avoid them. Ideal for HR directors and HIM directors, this video explores real-life scenarios and outlines practical security techniques.

For more information, contact:

Opus Communications, PO Box 1168, Marblehead, MA 01945
Telephone: 800/650-6787 or 781/639-1872
Fax: 800/639-8511 or 781/639-2982
E-mail: customer_service@opuscomm.com

Visit the Opus Communications World Wide Web site: *www.opuscomm.com*